FIRESIDE

Also by Christiaan Barnard

The Body Machine (Consulting Editor)
One Life
In the Night Season
South Africa: Sharp Dissection
*Good Life, Good Death: A Doctor's Case for
  Euthanasia and Suicide*

Christiaan Barnard's PROGRAM for LIVING with ARTHRITIS

by Christiaan Barnard
with Peter Evans

A FIRESIDE BOOK

PUBLISHED BY SIMON & SCHUSTER, INC.
NEW YORK

This book was devised and produced by Multimedia Publications (UK) Ltd

Editor: Peter Evans
Illustrations: Multimedia Publications (UK) Ltd

First published in Great Britain in 1984 by Michael Joseph Ltd

Library of Congress Cataloging in Publication Data
Barnard, Christiaan,
Christiaan Barnard's Program for living with arthritis.
"A Fireside book."
Bibliography: p.
Includes index.
1. Rheumatoid arthritis. 2. Barnard, Christiaan,
1922-   . 3. Rheumatoid arthritis—Patients—South
Africa—Biography. I. Title.
RC933.B343   1984   616.7'22   83-20264
ISBN 0-671-47052-3

Acknowledgments

The quotations in this book are reproduced by kind permission of the following:

George Allen & Unwin, London / Stein & Day, New York / J. Gomez: *How Not to Die Young* (1973);

Arthritis and Rheumatism Council / magazine contributors: J.S. Calnan, J. Charnley, A.S. Dixon, F. Dudley Hart, A. Hill, F. Mann;

Arthritis Foundation, USA: *Arthritis: Diet and Nutrition—Facts to Consider* (1983).

British Broadcasting Corporation; British Broadcasting Corporation / M. Freeman (Bone and Joint Institute) / M. Mason;

British Medical Journal / Ed. S. Lock / F. Dudley Hart (vol. 1, p. 763, 1976);

Martin Dunitz, London / F. Dudley Hart: *Overcoming Arthritis* (1981);

Granada Publishing, London / C.H. Dong and J. Banks: *New Hope for the Arthritic* (1980); *The Arthritic's Cookbook* (1983); Granada Publishing, London / J.H. Fries: *Arthritis and How to Cope With It* (1980);

Michael Joseph, London / Eds. O. Gillie, C. Haddon and D. Mercer: *The Sunday Times New Book of Body Maintenance* (1982);

Lancet / F. Dudley Hart, R.T. Taylor and E.C. Huskisson (vol. 1, p. 881, 1970);

Medical News;

New England Journal of Medicine / B.L. Koczin *et al.* (vol. 305, p. 969, 1981);

A.D. Peters / P. Wingate: *The Penguin Medical Encyclopedia:* (1972);

Practitioner / R.G. Gibson, S.L.M. Gibson, V. Conway and P. Chapell: *Perna canaliculus* in the treatment of arthritis (Septembere 1980);

Routledge & Kegan Paul, London / S. Hooker: *Caring for the Elderly* (1976);

Thames Television, London: *How to Last a Lifetime* (1983);

Charles C. Thomas, Illinois / R.H. Rahe: *Psychotropic Drug Response— Advances in Prediction* (1969) Eds. P.R.A. May and J.R. Whittenborn.

Contents

1   Where There's Life . . .   11

2   What Is Arthritis?   17

3   Treatment with Drugs   47

4   Keys to Self-Management   61

5   Spare-Parts Operations and Other Surgical Treatments   67

6   Living with Pain   77

7   Tips for Easier Living   87

8   Alternative Therapies   97

9   Arthritis and Stress: A Personal Dimension   115

10 Diet and Exercise   123

11 Looking Ahead: Arthritis Research   141

12 Some Reflections   147

    Bibliography   149

    Index   151

Christiaan
Barnard's
PROGRAM
for **LIVING**
with **ARTHRITIS**

WHERE THERE'S LIFE . . . 1

When Louis Washkansky became the world's first heart-transplant patient in 1967, I and my dedicated team of doctors and nurses had not only given that large, amiable man a new pump for circulating blood through his body. We had given him something perhaps more precious, without which life, in sickness or in health, is hardly worth living. We had given him that most vital commodity, hope.

Throughout my career, even before I began to perform heart-transplant operations, I had felt this need to open the door of hope to people who were hemmed in by fear or worry or despair. Perhaps it was what motivated me to become a doctor in the first place. But it was not until 1956, when I was a junior member of the surgical staff of the University of Minnesota, that I fully appreciated how important it is to have some light at the end of the tunnel. For it was in that year that I was diagnosed as having arthritis.

Imagine what this meant to me. I was a young, aspiring surgeon with a fast-developing expertise in the intricacies of open-heart surgery, and especially the possibilities of transplanting a new, healthy organ from one body to another. All surgery is physically as well as mentally demanding, imposing enormous strains on the surgeon as he stands for long periods carrying out delicate manipulations. With heart transplants there are added complications. For a start, the operations are performed with the aid of a battery of high-technology instruments of different kinds, all of which have to be monitored constantly to ensure that the right fluids are being delivered in the correct amounts, or that readings have not moved into the danger zone. Secondly, in transplant surgery you really have two "patients": the person whom you are fighting to save, and the precious heart, which must remain viable. In this complex medical setting, populated by large teams of surgeons, physicians, anesthetists, nurses, and auxiliaries, one needs to perform with maximum efficiency—which is not so simple when pain is crippling one's feet and legs, and one's hands are swollen and sore in practically every joint.

All this I could imagine so easily on that fateful day that my arthritis was diagnosed. And yet I was not without hope. Faced with the possible curtailment of my career before it had really lifted off, I still had something to cling to—a glimmer of optimism in the gloom. Let me explain how that came about.

In December 1955 I had gone from South Africa to the United States to take the job in Minnesota. This was a new experience for me because it was the first time that I had seen and been able to touch snow. In South Africa we rarely got snow in the city or the town. Snow is something found only up in the mountain peaks. Now, whether this change of climate had anything to do with what followed is hard to say. Before that, I had got interested in ice skating, but as I earned only two hundred dollars a month, I couldn't afford to buy skates, so I borrowed a pair from a friend, John Perry, who worked with me. The skates were rather narrow for my feet, and I remember that after going out skating one day, next morning I woke up with tremendous pain and soreness in my right foot. When I went in to work at the hospital, I talked to friends about the pain, and they said I probably had a fracture from the skating. I didn't take much notice of it, but then the foot became very swollen, and at the same time I developed a pain in my hands, especially my right hand. That, too, became swollen, so I realized it must be something other than a fracture.

In those days I was in general surgery, and because it was very difficult standing in an operating room for many hours with a painful foot, I went to the head of our department, the surgery professor, to speak to him about what I should do. As it turned out, I only saw his secretary, who said I should put my hands and feet in warm water, then put them in cold water, and that would probably stop the inflammation. This I tried for a few weeks, but to no avail. I then started wearing special shoes to try to ease the pain during periods of standing.

My hands, at that stage, were not in such a bad condition, but eventually the pain and swelling got so severe that I felt I had to see a rheumatologist. I went to the famous Mayo Clinic at the University of Minnesota, where the consultant examined me, did some blood tests, and then called me in and said: "Dr. Barnard, you are suffering from rheumatoid arthritis. But there's one thing in your favor—you are serum negative, and therefore it's very unlikely that you will ever be crippled by your arthritis."

Now, it is interesting that those words probably saved me, because when he told me that I had rheumatoid arthritis I immediately thought back to the first patient I ever examined and had to write up as a case history when I was a student in my fourth year of medical school in South Africa. This patient was a woman in her sixties who was totally bedridden with rheumatoid arthritis. She could hardly use her hands or her feet at all, and they were grossly deformed. So you can imagine that when the doctor at the Mayo Clinic told me I had rheumatoid arthritis, immediately a picture of this woman flashed through my mind and I thought to myself, "Oh, my God, here I am a young man who wants to become a surgeon, and with hands like that it would be totally impossible." But when this doctor told me my serum factor was negative (more on this later) and that I would probably never become actually crippled with arthritis, this acted as a tremendous encouragement to me. How important it is, when a doctor tells a patient of a disease that could permanently disable him or could be terminal, to leave a little bit of hope for the sufferer—even if the doctor feels deep down that the hope is very slight or that there is none at all.

That night I returned to the little room where I was staying and thought of what would now be the next step. Funnily enough, the first thing that occurred to me was to have my hands insured so that if anything should happen to me my family would be taken care of. (I was then married to my first wife, and we had two children.) I had read that some actresses insure their legs or their faces or even their voices for up to a million dollars, so I thought maybe I could have my hands insured for a million dollars. The problem was that if I went to insurers with such a proposition, I would have to lie. I would have to tell them that there was nothing wrong with my hands or feet, otherwise they would refuse to insure them. After thinking things over, I eventually decided to forget about the insurance and just see how things went on. So that is really how my long association with arthritis started.

At least, that is how it began for me in adult life. Certainly as a little boy growing up in Beaufort West, South Africa, I used to get odd aches and pains in the joints, sometimes severe enough to keep me awake at night. This condition was always diagnosed as "growing pains." Whether it was the forerunner of rheumatoid arthritis I am not sure. My father, who usually treated our family for minor ailments, would go down to our garden and take some green leaves from a bush, crush them, and pour hot water on them, leaving the mixture overnight. The next day I had to drink a cupful of the extract of these leaves. It was terribly bitter and usually gave me cramps and severe diarrhea, but somehow the pains in my joints disappeared after I took this remedy. These days, being constantly in pain, I often think I should go back to the garden of my youth and look for that bush with the green leaves.

As we shall see later in this book, there is some evidence that hereditary factors play a role in some forms of arthritis. One can inherit a set of genes from one's parents which somehow predispose toward the condition. Simply put, this means that arthritis appears to run in families. But I had four brothers, and none developed the disease. Nor were my parents sufferers. My father lived to the age of eighty-five and died of a lymphoma; my mother lived to the age of ninety-five and died from a stroke. True, my mother, in common with many elderly people, did complain of painful hands and joints during the later years of her life, but there was never any evidence of actual arthritis. So in my case I tend to rule out the genetic factor.

Let's go back again to those early years in Minneapolis. After the rheumatoid arthritis was diagnosed, I continued as a surgeon. Initially my hands were not severely affected. My chief concern was my feet, especially my right foot, which is really the only part of my body that has what you might call a deformity. (Since that time I have always been very shy about showing people my feet, especially my right foot. Conversely, I always admire beautiful feet, especially women's.) Arthritis apart, I continued to work hard—so hard that I established something of a record at the University of Minnesota. Within the short space of two and a half years, I completed a master's degree in science and a doctorate in philosophy, both of which involved writing a thesis. At the same time, though heaven knows where the time came from, I started to perform open-heart surgery, working up to eighteen hours a day. I spent very long stretches in the operating room, as even a simple procedure such as the closure of an atrial septal defect (a hole between the upper chambers of the heart) could take a whole day. The patient would be wheeled out late in the afternoon, but the medical team would be involved in post-op duties, which went on into the night. As the chief resident, I had to stay there the whole night. Yet even with my physical disability, I was able to tolerate these long hours of work and the intense strain, both physical and emotional. I cannot really remember, except for the sore hands and the difficulty I had in walking and standing, that I was really hampered by the arthritis.

Eventually I got metatarsal bars for my shoes, which I used in the operating room to take the weight off the metatarsal joints. That helped me a bit. But my appetite for work was voracious, pain or no pain. Could I have subconsciously thought that I might have a limited life span and thus developed the tremendous drive and determination to achieve as much as I did in those grueling two and a half years?

I returned to South Africa in 1958, bringing with me all the various components of a heart-lung machine. The head of the department of surgery at Cape Town's Groote Schur was keen for me to do open-heart surgery, because although the surgeons there had attempted it while I was in Minneapolis, the operation was a total disaster. I then started a laboratory, working on an oxygenator and training the team to run it while preparing for the program of open-heart surgery.

One day, when we were anesthetizing a dog, the animal bit me in the leg. Although I applied disinfectant, the wound became infected, producing a tremendous flare-up of my arthritis. For the first time my hands became so painful that I found it difficult to put on surgical gloves, and again the thought came to me that here I was at the beginning of a great career with an ailment that could end it all overnight. Once more the image of the deformed old woman with the gnarled fingers came back to me. But fortunately this exacerbation of my arthritis (whether it was due to the dog bite I am not sure) lasted only for a short while, so I found that I had problems only with my feet, not with my hands. No other joints were affected during that period.

The first open-heart operation I did with the heart-lung machine was a tremendous experience, stimulating but very stressful emotionally because not only did I have to perform the operation itself but I had to keep an eye on the heart-lung machine. When I and my assistants started the operation, I helped them open the chest and connect the patient to the machine. Then I unscrubbed quickly and helped the technicians to set the machine running. Then I ran back to help the surgeons to operate. Fortunately, it was an easy operation, which we were able to complete successfully, on a patient by the name of Joan Pick, who is still alive today. But for all the bustle of that and similar operations, my arthritis did not really affect me greatly. There were times when I was largely free of symptoms, and then out of the blue I would get a severe attack, mainly in one joint and not so often in my hands. Sometimes it was in the hip joints, sometimes in the knee, most often in the feet. Virtually within a few minutes it would flare up, the joint would become very swollen and painful, and then the episode would be over as quickly.

It would be a lie if I told you that at any stage these recurrent pains really seriously affected my work as a surgeon, but the arthritis *was* affecting me and interfering not so much with my surgery as with the auxiliary work a heart surgeon needs to do. In heart-lung surgery one has to push plastic tubes over connectors, and I remember that around 1967, not long before I did the first transplant, I started finding it difficult to push these tubes over the connectors, and I always asked my assistant to do it. Now, when we were preparing for the first heart transplant, I cannot remember having any problems with arthritis, nor during the transplant itself. Maybe I was so excited in the charged atmosphere that I find it difficult to remember. What I do recall is Louis Washkansky's death, eighteen days after the transplant. I was whisked off to the United States to do a television program, *Face the Nation*. I spent Christmas Day in the States and came back around the first few days of 1968. Immediately on my arrival, the British doctor Philip Blaiberg was ready for a heart transplant. Fortunately, there was also a suitable donor, so I had to operate on Dr. Blaiberg that night. I had difficulty during that operation because my hands and fingers were stiff and painful, terribly so as I was tying the sutures. But the operation was very successful, and Dr. Blaiberg was the first patient to have a transplant operation and leave the hospital. (He lived eighteen months after the transplant.)

As I now look back more than twenty years to the onset of my arthritis, I well remember the pattern. Life was full, even hectic: an endless round of work punctuated by rewards and, in the case of the early transplant successes, great excitement. There were times, and still are, when the pain was extreme, but somehow I managed to cope. What was my formula? Was I driven on by the need to realize my ambitions as a doctor and a scientist—what a psychologist would call "positive reinforcement"? Or was I motivated by the memory of that unfortunate woman of my student days? Was she my "aversion therapy"? Actually, when you think about it, it hardly matters which. Whether for positive or negative reasons, I was able to live with, if not master, my disability, hold on to a hope of succeeding or at least of not failing, of being able to continue in some sort of fashion. That hope is still there, and I want to share it with you in this book.

To do so I shall begin by switching roles. You have heard a little about the way I became a patient. In the next chapter I will be putting on my doctor's white coat to take a general look at the whole range of medical conditions we lump, a little crudely, under the heading "arthritis."

WHAT IS ARTHRITIS? 2

For the most part, people really only become interested in their bodies when something goes wrong. That is understandable. After all, if you jump in your car and it pulls away smoothly, corners properly, and brakes comfortably, you do not think it necessary to open the hood or check the chassis for faults. The working of your body, like that of your car, is easily forgotten if it gives you no trouble. Yet, to take the analogy one stage further, if the car does develop a mechanical fault and you want to put it right, you have to understand at least the basics of the system you are trying to remedy. Otherwise you could do more harm than good when you come to "rectify" the matter. Even if you put your car in the hands of a good mechanic—the automobile doctor—it would still pay you to know how the car works. You will know straightaway whether the repair has been competently and successfully carried out, and you'll be better able to spot trouble the second time around.

Similarly, if you are troubled with arthritis, you should know something about the basic mechanics of the system that has been malfunctioning. You will be better informed when talking with your doctor, more responsive to the treatments he will offer you, attuned to any danger signals, and most important of all, armed with a feeling of being at least partially in control of your situation.

So let's have a brief look under the hood, as it were, at the whole question of how normal joints are constructed, how they work, and then what happens to them when attacked by disease.

JOINTS AND HOW THEY WORK

A joint is the point of articulation (bending) between two bones. There are several types of joints: *fibrous* joints, such as the lower end of the shin bone where it meets the ankle; *cartilage*, as in the spine, where a disk of cartilage lies between the vertebrae; and *true* joints—the overwhelming majority—of which there are 187 in the human body, such as those in the

17

knees, fingers, and wrists. Although things can go wrong with any of these three types of joints, it is the last that mainly interests us simply because it is so common. The diagram shows how it is put together.

The true joint is a fairly complex piece of bodily engineering. The two facing bones are both capped with a layer of cartilage, a tough, gristlelike material, white in color and smooth in texture. The space around the joint, which is enclosed within the thin *synovial membrane,* and a tough *capsule* that holds the whole lot together, is filled with a lubricating fluid called *synovial fluid.* Tendons, too, help to hold muscle to bone, thereby keeping the joint together, while little pockets of fluid—the *bursae*—lie between muscles or muscles and tendons to lubricate body tissues that move across each other.

When you bend a finger, arm, or knee unaffected by joint disease, this beautifully engineered system works to perfection. The joint bends and straightens with a silkiness and lack of friction that mechanical engineers have been striving to achieve for centuries. What is more, the gristly cartilage acts as a shock absorber when you run downstairs, while the body generates, under normal circumstances, an endless supply of fresh synovial fluid to keep the bones moving smoothly. It is a self-contained, self-renewing system that will usually heal itself after injury.

A normal joint

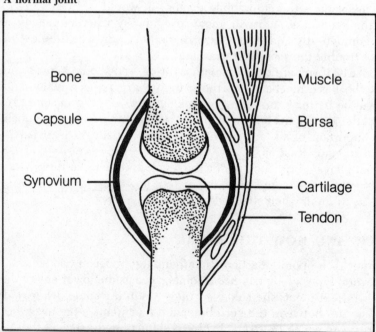

Some joints are more complex than others. Think, for example, of the shoulder joints when a tennis player throws up the ball to serve. The upper arm bone (humerus) moves on the shoulder blade. The shoulder blade moves on the ribs, and the collarbone (clavicle) moves on the shoulder blade. In fact, that tennis serve is calling into play three separate joints on the shoulder, not to mention elbow and hand movements. Or consider the joints in the spine as an Olympic gymnast carries out a breathtaking sequence of maneuvers on the beam. Here each separate bone in the back—each of the twenty-four vertebrae—moves on an intervertebral disk as the spine is flexed forward, backward, and from side to side. Again, considerable shock is put on the joints as a delicate cartwheel gives way to a violent handspring, ending with a triumphant two-footed landing. But with the spine it is not only the joint mechanism that has to be protected, for the nerves of the spinal cord run down a channel in the vertebrae, and if those are damaged, a superb athlete would become a paralyzed cripple.

You can see from this brief look at just two kinds of joints how complicated those juncture points can be—and how remarkably well they function, day in and day out, despite the colossal stresses, pressures, and strains we impose on them. You do not need to be a tennis player or gymnast to appreciate that.

WHAT IS ARTHRITIS?

What goes wrong when one contracts arthritis? Well, first of all, I am afraid that term "arthritis," though useful, is a bit misleading. The -itis part means "inflammation," so strictly speaking "arthritis" should be applied only to inflamed joints, whereas we tend to apply it to all joint diseases. There are certainly over 100 of these conditions involving joints (possibly over 180, depending on how you do your calculations), not all of which are arthritis. In fact, the degenerative condition known as osteoarthritis is misnamed because this really is an *arthrosis* (wear and tear in the joint). Then there are joint diseases under the heading of *arthropathy*, which can be inflammatory or degenerative. All very confusing, isn't it? Throughout this book I will stick with "arthritis" as a general rule, but for the sake of accuracy I will adopt the term "osteoarthrosis" instead of the more commonly used "osteoarthritis."

On, then, to these 100-odd joint diseases. We can categorize them in a number of ways, but I find it most helpful to think of the following six headings.

1. SYNOVITIS OR INFLAMMATORY DISEASE occurs when the synovial membrane, that thin layer of tissue which manufactures the lubricant synovial fluid, becomes red, swollen, and thick, forming folds. The result is a

joint with the classic symptoms of inflammation, known by the Latin words *calor* (heat), *dolor* (pain), *tumor* (swelling), and *rubor* (redness). The inflammation has two effects. First, swelling and pain; second, deformity in the joint by destroying its internal tissue. These symptoms are all highly familiar to me, as rheumatoid arthritis is the best-known disease in the synovitis group.

2. DEGENERATIVE DISEASE, of which osteoarthrosis is the best-known example, occurs when the cartilage over the bone ends gradually deteriorates with time, becoming worn and soft and flaking away from the bone. At its most extreme the cartilage disappears altogether so that bone rubs on bone. The result is stiff, painful joints. This is the "wear and tear" form of arthritis, most prevalent among older folks, although it can affect the young as well, as we shall see shortly.

3. INFECTIOUS DISEASES, caused by the presence of bacteria in the fluid of the joint, may strike one at any age. Various microorganisms can be implicated, such as staphylococcus or even gonococcus (which causes gonorrhea).

4. LIGAMENT AND TENDON PROBLEMS lead to joint pains where the ligaments and tendons join to the bone. Men are more prone than women, and the most common condition is the so-called poker back, or ankylosing spondylitis.

5. CRYSTAL INFLAMMATION is a form of arthritis in which the joint space becomes occupied by tiny crystals caused by an excess of uric acid in the body. Once the crystals set, they trigger off some of the most excruciating joint pain you can imagine, the most severe form of the condition being gout. I recall many a comedy sketch in which a crusty old gentleman with gout gets his heavily bandaged foot repeatedly knocked about. How odd it is that we make fun of chronic pain—until we experience it.

6. OTHER CONDITIONS include soft-tissue damage and a wide range of problems that are not strictly arthritic at all, such as muscle inflammation and injuries to tendons, ligaments, capsules, or bursae that cause tennis elbow, housemaid's knee, frozen shoulders, fibrositis, and so on. Often a minor strain will produce some of these, and, though painful, they usually disappear after a time. They are not really joint diseases in the manner of rheumatoid arthritis or osteoarthrosis.

These, then, are my six categories of arthritis. Let us now look a bit more closely at each of them, beginning with synovitis and especially rheumatoid arthritis, sometimes called "true arthritis."

RHEUMATOID ARTHRITIS

It is no exaggeration to describe rheumatoid arthritis (RA) as a disease affecting literally millions of sufferers worldwide. In the United States alone, for example, it has been estimated that 6.5 million people have the disease. Moreover, it is said that five times that number will contract RA at some time in their lives. For reasons that I will discuss later, the majority of these—three-quarters, in fact—are women. So numerous are arthritis sufferers, in fact, that I have often thought that my talents as a doctor might have been better deployed in rheumatology than in heart surgery. There would have been less glamour attached to it, but I would have helped more people. Anyway, my RA began in earnest in middle age, which is fairly typical, though there is a form called juvenile rheumatoid arthritis. (This is somewhat different from the adult version, and I will return to it a little later.)

The fact that RA combines both arthritis and rheumatoid symptoms may suggest that this is a joint condition brought on by cold and damp conditions, like colds and flu. In truth this is not the case. RA occurs as freely in hot countries like the West Indies or my native South Africa as it does

Changes in a joint caused by rheumatoid arthritis: (1) swollen joint and inflamed synovium; (2) erosion of cartilage; (3) loss of cartilage and erosion of bone

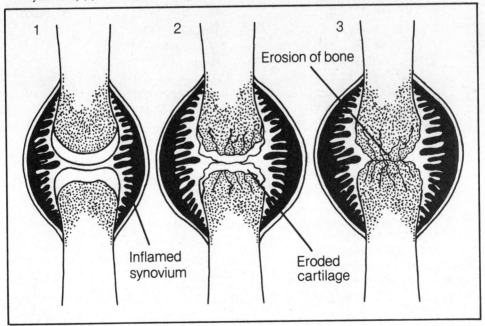

in the U.K., the U.S.A., or the U.S.S.R. The *rheum* element refers more to the stiffness, aches, and pains in the body that accompany the joint problems—a bit like the overall bodily symptoms of a raging bout of influenza.

That said, however, there are a few environmental curiosities. No population in the world seems exempt from RA, but research has shown that Eskimos and rural Negroes, for reasons as yet not understood, do have a degree of immunity. Even more fascinating, perhaps, is the finding among the African Bantu people who move into towns from the country. As rural dwellers, they have a slightly lower susceptibility than average. Once they are in the big city, the prevalence of RA among the Bantu rises to become no different, say, from that found in Britain. The same thing happens, incidentally, with coronary heart disease among Bantu moving into towns. What accounts for this town-country disparity? Fresh air? Less stress? Different diet? A combination of all three, together with some other less obvious factors? Or is it just an epidemiological quirk, a freak with no meaning at all? We can but wonder.

Many people would guess that the stress factor is the key, pointing out that RA appears, like coronary heart disease, to be a "disease of civilization." It looks as if it has increased substantially in modern times. Yet, when you dig a little deeper, you find that RA has a longer history than we tend to ascribe to it. Study of the ancient skeletons of Mexican Indians has revealed bone changes that could be due to arthritis, thousands of years ago. Then quite recently, four arthritis experts, an American and three Belgians, suggested that there is firm evidence for RA being in existence for at least 350 years. Theirs was an ingenious piece of medical detective work which began from the study of pictures painted by the great Flemish artist Rubens (1577–1640) in the last thirty years of his life. They found that individuals in the portraits showed the swollen hands and wrist joints familiar to today's sufferers, like myself. And the later the paintings, the worse the joints seem to become. Could the pictures be a reflection of Rubens's own arthritis? And could the chronological deterioration be paralleled by the artist's own hands? More recently there has been evidence that other painters, such as Renoir, tended to depict subjects with increasingly misshapen hands as their own disease progressed. If Rubens did the same, then his priceless works of art are also a vividly detailed case history of the first authenticated individual in medical science to suffer from RA—centuries before the stress-inducing world of the Industrial Revolution dramatically changed patterns of disease.

If not stress, then what does cause rheumatoid arthritis? Is one perhaps born with a genetically determined tendency toward the disease? Well, as I said earlier, in my own case RA did not seem to run in my family. My mother's hand joints became painful in her later years, probably as a result of life's wear and tear. So that would make her joint problems osteo, not rheumatoid. And remember that, apart from the usual run of childhood aches and pains, I never really became a "sufferer" from RA until middle age. If I did inherit the tendency, it was a long time expressing itself.

However, as with most topics in medicine, the hereditary element in RA is not an open-and-shut issue. Some doctors state that it is most definitely *not* an inherited disease, while others reason that our genes determine all aspects of our physical makeup, so they must to some extent, however small, be implicated in any illnesses to which we succumb. Thinking about this apparent contradiction led me to look at some of the current research in medical genetics that has a bearing on joint disease. And what I discovered gave me food for thought.

One of the most fascinating items to emerge was the project carried out by a British scientist, John Woodrow, at Liverpool University in 1981. Together with doctors in the English cities of Leicester and Coventry, Professor Woodrow appears to have identified the actual genes which pass on an increased tendency to RA from one generation to the next. What attracted me to Professor Woodrow's work in the first place, incidentally, was the fact that it has its roots in one of my own central preoccupations, tissue typing. When a heart-transplant candidate is being matched with a possible donor, it is vital that the tissue types of each be as close as possible, so that the donated heart will continue to be viable within the host body. Now, doctors know that there are around fifty tissue-type antigens— chemical elements on the outside surfaces of living cells which distinguish one person (or type) from another. In heart-transplant surgery, problems often arise after the operation when those antigens are simply not in harmony.

Professor Woodrow knew that the tissue-type factor called DR4 appeared to be involved in RA, because research on three different racial groups—American Negroes, Caucasians, and Japanese—had demonstrated that people with DR4 factor in their bloodstream were three or even four times more likely to contract RA than people without DR4. Professor Woodrow and his team studied the relationship between DR4 and rheumatoid arthritis in a white English population and again found that DR4 seemed to point to increased susceptibility.

However, when the researchers went on to investigate the same relationship among Asian Indians, they found not DR4 as the culprit but another tissue-type factor, DR1. Again, people with this factor in the blood were much more likely than average to contract the disease.

Putting both findings together, a picture emerges something like this. DR4 and DR1 are determined by two different genes, but both are on the same chromosome. It seems as if all the tissue-type-factor genes are situated close to one another on the same chromosome, from which they send

out their coded instructions to each cell to manufacture the relevant antigens. Thus, within a simple chromosome lies the genetic information to
determine susceptibility to arthritis of the rheumatoid variety. And the
structure of genes and chromosomes is in turn determined by heredity.
Among identical twins, who possess identical genes, there is a far higher
risk that both will develop the disease than in nonidentical twins. But not,
interestingly enough, a 100 percent overlap. So clearly there are factors
operating other than the genetic.

There are two other main theories to explain the onset of RA. One is
that the condition is caused by a defect in the body's immune system
known as autoimmune disease. Normally the immune system is an important part of our natural defense mechanism against infection. We, like all
other animals, have constantly to ward off the unwelcome advances of a
whole list of invasive organisms in the form of microbes trying to use our
bodies as a feeding and breeding ground. Under normal circumstances we
do this by mobilizing special cells that attack the invaders. For example,
if a bacterium were to enter a wound, the body would generate armies of
special white blood cells that act as phagocytes, engulfing and destroying
any bacteria in the vicinity. We are thus all in possession of a huge private
army of antibodies, specifically designed to recognize, hone in on, and
attack invasive microbes (antigens).

So far, so good. But this superb civil defense organization will sometimes break down. It happens, for example, with an allergy when the body
forms antibodies against perfectly harmless substances such as pollen and
behaves as if it were a potentially dangerous bacterium. This is the im-
munological basis of hay fever.

Similarly, there is a whole group of diseases in which the body forms
antibodies, not against any foreign matter, but against itself. It treats its
own tissue as antigenic and, as it were, declares civil war on itself—"hat-
ing itself," as it is sometimes described. Among the illnesses possibly due
to this autoimmune response are pernicious anemia, kidney disease, ul-
cerative colitis (inflamed intestinal lining), and—so some researchers believe—rheumatoid arthritis.

Once more, I find this an interesting thought because it ties in with my
own work on organ transplantation. To prevent rejection of a donor organ,
the doctors have to inject a patient with drugs to damp down his immune
responses, thereby preventing his natural defenses from ousting the "foreign" heart. If RA is an autoimmune disease, then some kind of drug treatment to suppress the immune system would seem to be a useful therapy.
Later I'll enlarge on this theme when I deal with the drugs currently
available for RA sufferers and the way in which I have used them.

Another theory as to what causes RA is that it is the effect of some as
yet unidentified virus. This, too, is an idea that I find perfectly reasonable,
especially in the light of some research carried out at the famous Guy's

Hospital in London by a group directed by Dr. Rodney Grahame. These scientists started from the well-known observation (first made about half a century ago) that people with German measles (rubella) often get the joint pains and swelling of arthritis, sometimes lasting for weeks. Now, rubella is caused by a virus that has the capacity to live in the body for months, even years, lying dormant, only to erupt long after it has initially infected the host. Could it be that arthritis is caused by the same virus? And could it also be that a childhood bout of German measles might produce joint problems far later in life? Well, Dr. Grahame found that five patients with a long history of arthritis did indeed show signs of rubella virus in the synovial fluid lubricating their joints. Curiously enough, though, three of the five had never suffered the usual German measles symptoms.

This could mean that arthritis is caused by a latent virus in people who have been subjected to an insidious hidden infection. Not for them the rashes and German measles that appear and disappear in childhood. Instead, they could be arthritis victims. It is a disturbing thought, isn't it, that any of us might be playing host to a virus that could proliferate by the million within our joints decades later? At the same time, if the rubella connection is a valid one, it may be that health authorities around the world should step up their vaccination programs in order to try to kill two medical birds with one stone.

My own view is that RA is, like coronary heart disease, one of those complex, multifactional diseases in which heredity, environment, infection, immune responses, and even psychological factors can and probably do all play their part, to a greater or lesser degree, depending on the individual. This may sound like a slightly euphemistic way of saying that doctors simply do not know yet what causes RA and can only offer us a few pieces of the jigsaw, and that is a criticism I will accept up to a point. On the other hand, it is no use trying to reduce to one explanation a disease that permits of many.

While we are on the subject of the various possible causes of rheumatoid arthritis, it occurs to me that this is an illness with a similarly baffling pattern of symptoms. Why is it, I have often wondered, that my arthritis is so capricious? One minute I feel severe pain as my hand or foot succumbs to a fierce bout of inflammation. The next I am in a natural, seemingly arbitrary period of remission. Of course, I try to do something about the pain and the inflammation; nevertheless there is a mysterious unpredictability—or so it seems—that makes nonsense of trying to anticipate the next onset. For me, as for any sufferer, this can be a nuisance, to say the least. There are some times in the day when one can face the prospect of pain, never a happy thought, more readily than others.

Interestingly enough, this variation in RA symptoms throughout the day has been studied scientifically by a distinguished team of rheumatologists and blood specialists in Britain and West Germany. They started from the experiences of arthritic patients who find that many signs and symptoms of the disease are worse at night and around the time of waking in the morning. At those times, sufferers tend to have stiffer joints and a weaker hand grip. Now, humans, in common with many other living organisms, have a natural timekeeping system, popularly known as a body clock but more correctly described as a circadian rhythm (from the Latin *circa*, "approximately," and *diem*, "day"). Many of our natural functions seem in no small part to be regulated by this inbuilt, twenty-four-hour chronometer, sleeping and waking being the most obvious.

The British and German team wondered whether variation in RA symptoms could in some way be dictated, or at least influenced, by a body-clock mechanism. Accordingly they chose ten hospital patients with RA and observed their symptoms over a twenty-four-hour period, taking blood samples and assessing pain and stiffness at regular intervals. When the results were analyzed, they found that joint stiffness and impaired grip strength were at their height between two and four A.M. and lowest at four P.M. Their first thought was that the immobility of patients at night causes an increase of fluid content in the joint tissues, but this they had to discount because patients who were confined to bed, and virtually immobile day *and* night, showed similar patterns of symptoms. Another explanation was that the inflammatory process itself—the biochemical abnormality in the bloodstream, as it were—is subject to diurnal variation, especially if a person is on a course of anti-inflammatory drugs, as those ten patients all were.

For my part, it is only in the last two years or so that I have experienced joint pain at night of such a severity as to keep me awake. But I do know that the early morning is often a critical time in many illnesses. The body seems to be at its lowest ebb. Indeed, many deaths in hospitals occur at this time, including that of Louis Washkansky, the first transplant patient, who finally succumbed in the early morning hours.

Whatever the explanation, it is certain that those sudden excruciating bursts of pain in the joints are not some punishment from on high, but a perfectly normal, if infuriating, pattern of events in RA, just like the pain-free phases afterward. If this variability is bewildering for the patient, by the way, it also does not help the doctor, because he has to make clinical assessments, say, of the usefulness of a drug he has prescribed at certain times of the day. It may be that he catches you at a good, or bad, time and therefore could be misled in his judgments.

Diagnosing RA and Predicting Its Outcome

As we saw earlier, swelling and pain—*tumor* and *dolor*—are the key symptoms of inflammatory diseases in general and arthritis in particular.

These are what eventually forced me to consult the rheumatologist at the Mayo Clinic. He carried out a number of tests before arriving at his unwelcome diagnosis, and it might be as well to run over these here so that you know what they are should you be at that stage of wondering: "Have I got it?"

Before doing so, however, you may like to do a preliminary check on yourself just to make sure that you are not being the overanxious sort who tends to mistake a transient pain in the foot due to too much standing on high heels for gout or something worse. Conversely, a simple test will convince you that you are not worrying unnecessarily and that the pain you are experiencing really does warrant further investigation. The celebrated arthritis expert Dr. Frank Dudley Hart puts it very nicely when he writes: "The unimaginative stoic will often put up uncomplainingly with what turns out later to be early rheumatoid arthritis, while the frightened introspective subject suffers the tortures of the damned from what turns out to be a simple bunion. Early symptoms of disease can often be misinterpreted badly, even by medical experts. What chance, therefore, can the uninformed patient have of getting it right?"

Well, what chance is there? Even a doctor can misinterpret the signs and symptoms, as I discovered when I began to develop a persistent cough a few years ago. This was accompanied by some of the classic signs of heart disease: shortness of breath, tiredness, and so on. Or maybe, I thought, I have lung cancer. Well, I struggled on for weeks with this wretched cough, until I finally consulted a doctor friend, who diagnosed asthma. Relief all around, and a further confirmation of the difficulties of knowing what is wrong. Anyway, here are a few typical signs of arthritis in the early stages.

1. Early-morning stiffness and pain
2. Tenderness of the bottoms and balls of the feet when walking
3. Swelling and soreness in fingers and wrists (These finger pains are often the first to appear, by the way.)
4. Restricted movement and swelling in shoulder, elbow, and knee joints (usually not in end finger joints)
5. A general run-down feeling, with loss of weight and/or appetite
6. The above symptoms last for at least six weeks.

When, eventually, I went to the Mayo Clinic, initially just with foot pains, the rheumatologist initiated a series of tests. But during his first examination he discussed the condition with me, asking about the six points listed above. It did not take him long, even before I was tested, to make his preliminary diagnosis. Nevertheless, off I went for laboratory tests to verify whether arthritis was indeed the culprit, how serious it was, and—the nagging worry that was burning away in my head—how would it progress in the future.

At the Mayo one receives the full battery of investigations. First a blood sample is taken so that the so-called *erythrocyte sedimentation rate* or ESR could be measured. Erythrocytes are red blood cells, which will settle in a column of blood in a glass tube. The faster they settle, the more active is a disease. Thus, ESR measurements are a kind of index of severity, especially of inflammatory illness, including RA and also, incidentally, rheumatic fever. A second test was the rheumatoid factor test or *latex fixation test*, which looks for the presence of the rheumatoid factor or antibody in the bloodstream. If the finding is serum positive, that bodes less well than serum negative, which was the case with my diagnosis. However, although that phrase "serum negative" helped me enormously by giving me hope, it may have been slightly illusory. It is not uncommon for a negative finding to give way to a positive one later on. It usually does so, in fact, because four out of five RA sufferers end up serum positive.

Apart from those two primary tests, the Mayo doctors also carried out other investigations. They drained off (aspirated) a little fluid from around the joints to study the inflammatory cells under the microscope, checking at the same time for the presence of an infective bacterium. They did an *antinuclear antibody* (ANA) test, a *total complement* test, and the *immunoelectrophoresis* test, all designed to show whether the joint problem was RA or one of several other conditions with superficially similar symptoms. There were also, of course, *x-ray examinations*, to see to what extent bones and cartilage had been damaged by the disease. In those early days they found nothing unusual, by the way, which is quite normal even when RA is very severe.

At the same time that the Mayo rheumatologist made his diagnosis, he also—urged on by me, I should add—offered his prognosis, saying that he thought my chances of being "crippled" by RA were relatively modest. I felt relieved, or perhaps "reprieved" would be more accurate, tempering my more pessimistic thoughts with the consolation that I was slightly privileged, if that is the right word, not to be destined to become an immobile invalid.

Actually I was, I soon found out, nothing special in this respect. The Mayo doctor went on to remind me that probably only one in six RA sufferers becomes crippled or deformed by the disease, and only one in ten progresses to a severe disability. Surveys have shown that the outlook for all RA sufferers is far from being bleak right across the board. Twenty percent—one in five—recover completely without any permanent joint incapacity. A further 20 percent recover with only minor abnormalities in the joints, while 50 percent experience continuing pain and inflammation in varying degrees of severity. In short, I and anyone else diagnosed as having RA have a fifty-fifty chance of being relatively untroubled by the condition in the future. And what will determine the outcome, in no small measure, is the treatment and management that are recommended and practiced. This was made plain to me at the Mayo, and that note of hope was music to my worried ears. But before we go on to the treatment of RA, this seems a good point at which to look in more detail at some of those other hundred or so arthritis ailments I listed earlier. If RA is your particular concern, and you have no other interest in things rheumatological, jump on to Chapter 3.

JUVENILE RHEUMATOID ARTHRITIS (JRA)

One last point, though, on RA. In my case the disease hit me in middle age. However, there is—surprisingly, you might think, if you associate arthritis with advancing years—a form of RA that affects children. Juvenile rheumatoid arthritis (JRA) is fortunately quite rare. Four out of five apparent "rheumatic" pains in children turn out to be something less serious. Nonetheless, JRA is estimated to affect about 12,000 children in the United Kingdom alone. So, on a worldwide scale, the problem is numerically not inconsiderable.

The term "juvenile rheumatoid arthritis" is a bit misleading, by the way, because it suggests that the symptoms, treatment, and outlook are very similar to the adult form. In fact, children with arthritis have problems quite different from those I have encountered, and their recovery prospects are much better than those of the adult. There are several forms of the condition among the young, but the one most people think of is what is sometimes called Still's disease, after the English physician G. F. Still, who described the symptoms at the famous Great Ormond Street Children's Hospital in London. The big difference between adult and juvenile forms is, as I have mentioned, that recovery prospects are much better for children. Seventy percent of those who contract arthritis in early life, even as very young children, make a good recovery. I have always regarded child patients as deserving a very special sort of care, so I shall say more on the subject of juvenile arthritis later on, in Chapter 7. Now on to those forms of arthritis other than RA which affect the adult. Just to remind you, apart from synovitis such as RA, the other forms of arthritis are:

degenerative arthritis (such as osteoarthrosis)
infectious arthritis
ligament and tendon arthritis
crystal arthritis (such as gout)
other types, including soft-tissue damage

We must put the degenerative forms at the top of our list because, of course, they embrace osteoarthrosis (OA), the kind of joint problem that the majority of people get as they grow older; it is practically the universal disease, you might say.

OSTEOARTHROSIS

Look at the diagram of cartilage degeneration, including the magnified section. You can clearly see how this tough, gristly material has literally worn away, allowing the bone to grind on the facing bone like a ball bearing wearing away its seating when it has been starved of lubricant. And this in a way is what is happening in the OA joint. The cartilage loses its elasticity and fails to provide a smooth seating for the bones of the joint. At its worst the cartilage wears away completely. Sometimes the unprotected bones, rubbing against each other, end up polishing their own surfaces, thereby easing the joint again. But for the most part, loss of cartilage is equal to loss of suppleness.

Virtually every medical reference describes OA as the outcome of life's general wear and tear. The most vulnerable are the joints that bear the biggest loads. The legs, hip, and spine, for example, may be subjected to abnormal stresses through bad posture or injury. A joint that has been operated on will be more prone than one that has not. And yet OA is not exclusively an "old man's disease." True, aching and stiffness in the joints are more likely to be a problem in middle age and beyond. True, the seventy-year-old is more likely to have knobby knee or finger joints than someone thirty years his or her junior. However, of the estimated five million OA sufferers in Britain (probably twice that in the U.S.), many are comparative youngsters, in their twenties and thirties.

A fascinating study carried out in England by Juliet Rogers, Iain Watt, and Paul Dieppe from Bristol Royal Infirmary showed that OA has been a problem in a wide age range for a very long time. Their evidence came from a collection of skeletons uncovered by archeologists excavating medieval and Saxon sites in the west of England. The bones were examined under x-rays, and it was seen that osteoarthrosis, especially of the hip and shoulder, was very common in the twenty- to fifty-year age range in Saxon and medieval England. In fact, arthritis generally was a problem. In writing up their results in the *British Medical Journal* (Dec. 19–26, 1981), the researchers expressed surprise at the particularly high incidence of OA. So often we regard "wear and tear" illnesses as diseases of civilization, but the three researchers were forced to conclude that "arthritis was as big a problem to our ancestors as it is now."

According to the consultant rheumatologist Dr. Anne Nicholls, the near universality of OA among the elderly does not prove that aging and wear and tear on their own are the cause of the disease. She points out that there appear to be racial differences in the incidence of the disease. It is, for example, high in the town of Leigh in Lancashire but low in the northern European town of Heinola in Finland. She also goes on to suggest that OA may have a metabolic basis in that people with certain metabolic disorders seem more prone to the arthritic condition. There is, further, a tendency for OA to affect relatives. Putting all the data together, then, Dr. Nicholls concludes that both the occurrence and distribution of OA may be genetically determined. Other, external factors of the wear-and-tear variety are clearly important, but to some degree (how far it is difficult to say) we seem to be born with a predisposition to OA. Long before we start putting stresses on our joints, the die is cast.

Hormones, too, seem to play a part. Generalized osteoarthrosis, it seems, is more common among women than men and will often begin to be a problem at around the menopause, the so-called change of life, when a variety of major hormonal events take place. It is as if the natural diminution of female hormones, signaling the end of the childbearing phase in a woman's life, provides a setting for joint problems to appear, especially if there is the added aggravation of even quite minor knocks and injuries.

Whatever the causes of OA—and in many cases I am inclined to think these are multifactional, a combination of several factors—the signs and symptoms are all too familiar as we look around us. How often have we seen an elderly person with knobby, enlarged finger joints? What happens is that hard knobs or nodes (known as Heberden's nodes) develop around the edges of a joint as the cartilage breaks down. In the beginning you

Cartilage degeneration: wearing out of the joint gristle

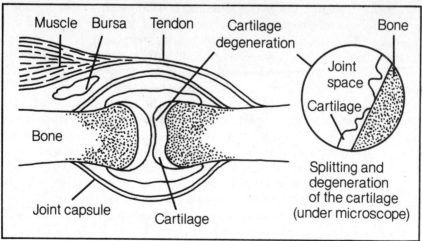

may just feel a bit of pricking or soreness in the end joints of the fingers, along with a little swelling and stiffness, but usually not severe pain. Your finger movements, though, may be less than perfect, especially on fine-detail tasks, and you may begin to notice that the tingling develops into a definite ache or pain if you have been using your hands vigorously, whether scrubbing floors or crashing through a dramatic passage of Beethoven on the piano. The sensations may develop as well at the base of the thumb. After a time the joint may become painful to the touch. The prickling has been succeeded by a very pronounced discomfort.

Over a period of years the nodes with their accompanying pain may spread to other finger joints, and indeed OA may set in elsewhere in the body. Sometimes (though rarely) in women of middle age a bony swelling will come and go over a period of a few weeks, not persisting to produce a permanent incapacity.

As we move from the hands to other parts of the body, the familiar characteristic symptoms are pain, stiffness, thickening of the joint, and loss of mobility, to a greater or lesser degree. The big toe, like the thumb, will become knobby at the base, usually not causing much pain but producing a problem if it begins to "drift" over the other toes (a condition called *hallux valgus*). At this point one may have to sacrifice a preference for relatively constricting shoes, especially high heels, in the interests of getting around unencumbered.

If one is lucky, OA might confine itself to thumbs, fingers, and big toes. In that case, in the words of Dr. Frank Dudley Hart, it is "a nuisance, but not serious, and like osteoarthritis in any other joint, does not affect your general health or your insurance policy." Nevertheless, Dr. Dudley Hart goes on to point out, "these nagging aches and pains can cause a considerable upset and interference with normal living and working." The good news is that although OA is the near-universal ailment, a chronic condition of widespread prevalence, it cripples only a few, and indeed only a minority will have to resort to any form of treatment for it.

Osteoarthrosis can, of course, affect joints other than in the hands and feet. The knee and its load-bearing region are vulnerable, again with thickening and stiffness, and may be a site where fluid accumulates—the graphically described condition of "water on the knee." One unfortunate result of the arthritic knee, apart from causing difficulty in walking, is that it can give the legs a bowed shape or, conversely, a knocked-kneed appearance. I can understand fully why people with one or the other of these symptoms feel stigmatized, if not downright angry. It is one thing to have one's appearance changed by a disease and quite another to have it distorted in such a way as to make the sufferer an unwilling figure of fun. For my part it has not been so much that fear as a feeling of sheer embarrassment. When I step out of my car in front of the hospital in the morning, I get anxious lest friends and colleagues catch me on a bad day, when I am walking particularly badly because of stiffness in my feet. It embarrasses me. To be frank, I have always been rather proud of my body, how I have been able to use it either in sport or at work as a surgeon. To be seen hobbling across the parking lot, up the stairs, or along the hospital corridors I find acutely painful in itself. So I put on a teeth-gritting act, smiling my way along, taking the stairs up four or five floors, and ignoring the elevator. That is the sort of length I would go to in order to avoid being pointed to or sniggered at—even though I know deep down that very few people would really react that way if they did see signs of my arthritis.

After years of attempting to maintain this sort of subterfuge, I can now take, as it were, a step back and look more dispassionately at my attitudes toward the outward signs of arthritis than I did during the early days. On balance, I probably exaggerated other people's reactions to my showing signs of illness and would recommend to anyone that they try not to hide too much. Not that you should, on being diagnosed, immediately throw in the towel and declare yourself an invalid from here on in. But come to terms with the inevitable.

In OA, for example, you may find that your hitherto unobtrusive knee-caps begin to produce a variety of odd noises—clicks and rubbing sounds. Those you may find more embarrassing than worrying, which is good to some extent because they are usually less ominous than they sound. But don't try to cover them up too much by keeping unduly still in company or by any other dodge of that kind. If you do, you may suffer in two ways. First, your embarrassment leads to resentment and bitterness, a feeling of being victimized. This is something I know a lot about, and it does you no good whatsoever. Second, it seems, paradoxically enough, to actually make the joint worse if you try to disguise symptoms. This probably has something to do with one's psychological makeup and how it affects one's pain threshold (which we will look at later).

Make no mistake about it. I am not saying that you should retreat into illness as soon as you feel your very first twinge of OA. But don't swing to the other extreme and live in a fantasy world of believing that you need never show your "weakness."

Suppose, for example, the disease affects your hip, another load-bearing joint which is prone to OA. As it progresses, it could mean that you feel more comfortable walking with a stick. Is that such a bad thing? When you think about it, a stick is just a mobility aid like a bus or a luggage cart. Of course, you could take the tougher option and walk to every destination, rain or shine, or struggle single-handedly with your suitcases. But it makes sense for the occasion to use an aid. Think of a walking stick in the same way—not as a badge of infirmity but as a means to an end, to be employed whenever and wherever it suits *you*.

How do you know whether your aching or painful joints indicate OA rather than, say, synovitis? Well, for a start, the pain tends to be local, and the symptoms specific. Most arthritics suffer from general feelings of being run down or out of sorts, especially when in repeated pain, but unlike the rheumatoid arthritis sufferer, the osteo patient will not generally feel aches and pains. Discomfort will tend to be confined to one or several specific joints.

Your doctor may consider that further investigation is called for, in which case the principal test is by x-ray. With x-rays it is possible to get some idea of the extent of deterioration in the mechanism of the joint—how much the joint space has narrowed, for example. But these pictures of the joint can be misleading in that aberrations in structure are more common than symptoms. In other words, you could take x-ray pictures of the joints of nonsufferers and still find something, strictly speaking, amiss. One thing of interest that does show up, though, is the presence of little bony growths, or *osteophytes*, which tend to develop where the cartilage has degenerated. The more numerous the osteophytes, the more cartilage has been lost.

As OA is very much a local degenerative condition, there is little to be gained from a blood test, except to rule out any other form of arthritis or indeed any other illness which is reflected in abnormalities in the bloodstream.

I said earlier that OA is likely to affect people who have for one reason or another placed unusual demands on their joints, as opposed to the general run of sufferers whose problem just seems to develop out of nowhere. Doctors sometimes make a distinction between this latter type of OA, calling it primary osteoarthrosis, implying that the original cause of the degenerative change is unknown, and the former type, dubbed secondary. If you have been involved in an accident or suffered any other kind of injury such as a fracture, this could initiate secondary OA, by damaging either the surfaces of the joint bones or their alignment with each other. Alternatively, you may have had the misfortune to be born with, say, a hip misalignment, which is self-aggravating. Or you may have contracted some form of disease that interferes with the mechanical efficiency of the normally smooth joint. In all these secondary cases, the most vulnerable regions are, again, those on which you make the highest demands. Joggers, for example, who run on hard surfaces seem to me to be asking for joint trouble. In fact, I am generally convinced of the joys of jogging, remembering the motto "Jogging is like a cold bath. You feel better when it's finished."

As an example of OA caused by misalignment, I can cite myself. I was once hit by a car; it came out of nowhere and knocked me clear across the road. Eleven of my ribs were broken, and my lung was pierced so that after I was treated at the hospital, I got into the habit of walking with a slight sideways stoop to reduce the discomfort. The habit stayed and so did the stoop. My spine responded to this newly adopted alignment by fixing itself out of its rightful position. This has led to posturally induced arthritic pains in the back. Remember, if you are forced temporarily to change your posture, revert to an upright carriage as soon as you can.

A word of caution here, whether you have or think you have primary or secondary OA. Using the joints in a strenuous fashion does not of itself necessarily cause or even predispose toward arthritis. Research on people whose job forces them to subject joints to severe stress has not come up with any clear-cut connection. So pain in a joint should definitely not be a cue for you to give up using it. Indeed, there is evidence that joint problems may be slightly more likely in those who are relatively inactive. Moderation, then, is called for, not renunciation.

INFECTIONS IN THE JOINT

The space between two joint bones can sometimes be invaded by infectious microorganisms in the form of bacteria. Indeed, practically every kind of bacterium known to medical science seems to be able to produce joint problems. The commonest are *staphylococcus* (staph for short), a spherical bacterium only 1/25,000 of an inch in diameter; *gonococcus*, better known as the organism that produces the sexually transmitted disease gonorrhea; and the *tubercle bacillus*, again better known for a different effect, namely as causing tuberculosis. To this list of chief protagonists can be added a number of others, including the *syphilis spirochete* and the *pneumococcus*, both usually associated with ailments other than arthritis.

The invasion of bacteria in the joint space is rapid and needs quick attention by means of antibiotics. If one of your joints swells in the space of a few hours to form a hot, red, painful, balloonlike area, seek medical help quickly. Not only can potent microbes permanently damage the joint, but they can spread to other parts of the body. It is of course difficult to avoid contracting infections in the first place. No amount of care and caution, even if you are a Howard Hughes, will protect you from every microbe floating around. But a rapid response to the first signs of infection is vital because, as Dr. Frank Dudley Hart puts it, "quick control of an infection in its early stages may make all the difference between a prolonged low-grade illness and a quick recovery."

Infection in the joint may arise as a by-product of infection elsewhere in the body, with a few dangerous bacteria being carried to the joint space by way of the bloodstream. In certain circumstances, some individuals are more ready prey to infectious bacteria than others—for example, a heart-transplant patient given a course of immunosuppressive drugs. But generally the comings and goings of bacteria seem a matter of chance.

The worst infectious arthritis I have ever witnessed was some years ago when I was a medical student; it was in the knee joint of a young man who was a keen rugby player. During one match, he was severely tackled and his opponent's teeth accidentally sank into his knee. This was before antibiotics, so a rampant infection set in unchecked. Eventually, the poor lad had to have his leg amputated as the damage was so severe.

With staph infections usually only one joint, perhaps the knee, wrist, elbow, hip, or ankle, will be affected; sometimes several. The infection will cause a high temperature and a general ill feeling. If such an infection is suspected, doctors will act quickly, for delay can be serious, even fatal. They will carry out blood tests to identify the offending organism as well as x-ray examinations to check for signs of joint damage.

It may come as some surprise to learn that the gonococcus organism can cause arthritis, but this is indeed the case. It may derive from an initial genital infection that is carried in the bloodstream to the joints. Most at risk are young women (ten times more so than men), who will often fail to notice any venereal infection in the very early stages, whereas men are alerted to it by penile discharges. Again, one or several joints may be infected: usually the knee, wrist, and ankle. What may also happen with gonococcal arthritis is that a few blisters appear on the skin. These are little surface outposts of bacteria which could signal a joint problem elsewhere.

One should act quickly if there is any discharge from the penis or va-

Infection of the joint space

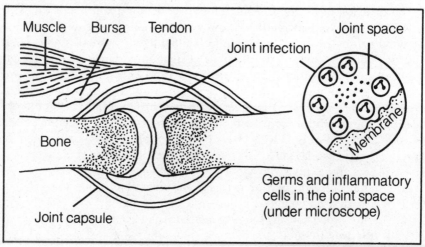

Muscle   Bursa   Tendon   Joint space
Joint infection
Bone
Joint capsule
Membrane
Germs and inflammatory cells in the joint space (under microscope)

gina, not only in order to curb venereal disease but to protect the joints. These joint infections are less serious than the staphylococcal types, usually leaving no permanent joint damage, provided they are quickly diagnosed and properly treated by antibiotics.

Do not automatically think that pains in the joints and symptoms such as urinary irregularities mean that you have contracted a sexually transmitted disease. I remember a few years after I had been diagnosed an arthritic I suddenly developed a urethral discharge. I was horrified because I thought I had developed gonorrhea. There was a certain amount of dysuria (pain in passing water) with it, too, but I was too scared to speak to anybody about it because it was such a disgrace. So I started using penicillin, because I thought that would cure the infection, but it didn't. It went on and on, and eventually I was so upset about it that I did consult a doctor. Well, it turned out to be urethritis—an inflamed urethra—a condition which one often gets with rheumatoid arthritis. (One can also get eye problems such as conjunctivitis.) In my case it was a happy ending, as the urethritis spontaneously disappeared after a while. But the moral of the story is: if you think you might have a gonococcal infection, see your doctor *now*.

Joint problems caused by the tuberculosis microbe are infrequent compared with those produced by staphylococcus or gonococcus. They also arise comparatively slowly, so that a knee or hip joint swells painfully over a period of weeks or months, not hours or days. Usually only one joint is affected, and the diagnosis is made by taking a sample of the surrounding fluid and culturing it to identify the bacterium. If there is any long-term damage to the joint, as indicated by x-ray examination, this, too, can take a long time to develop. Prompt treatment is vital, though, to avoid the risk of permanent disability.

LIGAMENT AND TENDON PROBLEMS (*Attachment Arthritis*)

This is a group of arthritic conditions that derive not so much from a malfunctioning specifically at the point where one bone meets another as from a problem with ligaments or tendons attached to the joint bones.

Ankylosing Spondylitis

The best-known and commonest form of attachment arthritis is ankylosing spondylitis (AS), sometimes called poker back. It predominantly affects young and middle-aged men (ten times more often than women). AS has been around for many hundreds of years. X-ray studies of the bones of Egyptian mummies have revealed signs of the typical changes associated with it, though curiously enough it is literally only within the last fifteen to twenty years that all rheumatologists have recognized it as a condition quite distinct from rheumatoid arthritis, which in many ways it resembles.

The trouble usually begins in the back. In fact, *spondylitis* means literally "inflammation of the joints in the spine" (*spondylos* is Greek for "vertebra"). Pains tend to occur in the sacroiliac joints between the sacrum and the pelvis (see diagram), where inflammation is localized in the bone ligaments and tendons. Many sufferers are often wrongly diagnosed in the early days as having a slipped disk and given an inappropriate form of treatment. Later, though, if AS progresses to become severe, it is easy to spot the sufferer. He has a rigid, painful spine, often bent like a question mark. He holds up his head with difficulty when walking, though his appearance is normal when he is seated.

Ankylosing spondylitis appears to have a genetic basis, for it tends to crop up in relatives of sufferers twenty times more frequently than in the general population. And again it shows some racial peculiarities. There is a high prevalence among certain American Indian tribes. It is unusual in the Japanese and appears to be virtually unknown among African Negroes.

The root of the problem, as I said earlier, lies in fibrous tissue attaching to the bone, and not (as in RA) in the synovial lining. Some joints, of which the sacroiliac joint is one, turn on fibers rather than a synovial lining, so the disease tends to be limited to these. With time the stiffness and pain in the lower back may spread to other joints. The typical sufferer might begin to feel discomfort further up the spine, sometimes in the chest when he coughs. It becomes painful to bend down to pick something up, and it is not uncommon for someone with AS to experience sharp pains in the joint in the chest which connects the two parts to the breastbone. In fact, more than one AS sufferer has mistakenly thought that this chest pain indicates a heart condition.

Possibly the worst symptom of AS is a psychological one, that of being trapped by the disease. As Dr. A. S. Dixon of the Royal National Hospital for Rheumatic Diseases in Bath, England, puts it: "Soon the sufferer describes a feeling of being locked in, imprisoned almost, with his own bones, and bed rest still seems to make things worse." The unluckier AS victims find the joint stiffness and pain spreading to the hips and other areas, including the fingers, until, in Dr. Dixon's graphic phrase, "In practical terms they become living statues." This is the gloomiest picture. Though very common and at times severe, AS will usually not prevent a person from working and taking an active part in life. The majority of AS sufferers, with some limitation, live quite normally.

So far as diagnosis is concerned, it may be some time—several years or even longer—before AS is recognized. Initially, it is, as you can imagine, quite easy for doctors to confuse it with lumbago, sciatica, or simply "aches

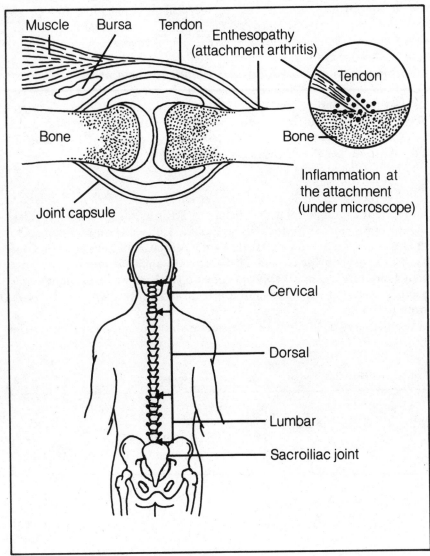

Ankylosing spondylitis: "poker back" disease. A normal backbone (*bottom*) can be affected in the same way as any movable joint (*top*).

and pains." And there are often no visible signs of the disease. One interesting and slightly surprising symptom, though, is an inflammation of the iris of the eye—iritis—which may occur from time to time. So if, in addition to back pain, stiffness, and a general feeling of being unwell, you develop a red eye, see your doctor and discuss rheumatological tests. These will usually consist of x-rays of the sacroiliac joints, which will show signs of the disease if it has been present for a couple of years. Also the sedimentation rate test will be carried out and abnormalities looked for, though often the rate is perfectly normal. In recent years a genetic test has also been coming into use. This is the so-called *HLA B-27 antigen blood test*, which can tell doctors whether a person has an inborn tendency toward AS. Only a tendency, mind you. A positive finding does not of itself prove that the disease is present.

Reiter's Disease

Another form of tendon and ligament arthritis, again most prevalent among young men, is Reiter's disease, named after a German army doctor who first described it during World War I. Although Reiter's is second only to AS in causing arthritis among young men and teenagers, it is in fact really quite rare. Again, it appears to be unusual among black populations. Again, it has a genetic basis, and the B-27 antigen test will usually prove positive.

What triggers off Reiter's disease seems to be an infection. This can be

Crystal arthritis: inflammation within the joint space

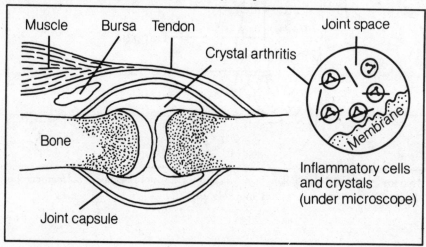

of a sexual nature or it can derive from certain forms of dysentery. But whatever the infective organism, the symptoms of arthritis seem to be associated with eye inflammation (conjunctivitis), discharges from the penis, and skin rashes.

Again, as with AS, the sacroiliac joints are vulnerable, as is the spine in general. However, pain and stiffness can be experienced elsewhere. Pain in the heel, for example, is quite common, as are distorted finger or toe joints.

Reiter's disease tends to come and go in episodes, sometimes only one or two with no recurrences. As with AS, the severity of the disease will range from mild and untroubling to extreme and, in a minority of cases, even crippling. In general terms, though, most sufferers manage to cope well.

CRYSTAL ARTHRITIS: GOUT

Visitors to the Cotswold hills of Britain are always struck by the charm of the place and its picturesque villages with evocative names: Bourton-on-the-Water and Stow-on-the-Wold are world-famous as beauty spots, and rightly so. Yet a few years ago, scientists from the British Arthritis and Rheumatism Council made a curious discovery. They had been called in by local doctors concerned about the number of people coming to them, especially females, with the symptoms of gout. For reasons that remain a mystery, gout in the Cotswolds is more prevalent than normal in the U.K. It could be that the local water supply or some other environmental factor is to blame—though no one was able to trace any such factor. Indeed, there was no association between gout and length of residence in the area, which did seem to argue against the theory of long-term exposure to environmental conditions. In short, here was a clear-cut finding that produced medical bafflement.

And yet gout is probably the form of arthritis about which most is known. It certainly has a long history, dating back to pre-Christian times. Traditionally it has been held to be a "superior" form of arthritis because it appears to be common among the high and the mighty, as witness this vignette from Dr. Collin H. Dong and Jane Banks in their book *New Hope for the Arthritic* (London: Granada, 1980): "A caricature of the gourmand King Henry VIII, seen in comic strips, is a picture description of gout that is worth ten thousand words. King Henry is shown as a fat, well groomed monarch sitting on a great chair with his leg bandaged and with a big, red, inflamed toe exposed, resting on a footstool. In one hand he holds a large rib of beef and in the other a mug of ale." Elsewhere we see bearded, crusty, gouty retired army colonels or self-indulgent landowning earls, their swollen feet swathed in bandages, treated usually as figures of fun as they sip yet another glass of port and complain of their aching feet.

What manner of disease, then, is gout? Is it confined to kings and castle owners with a taste for too much food and especially drink? Well, clearly not, if the Cotswold survey is anything to go by, nor if we look a bit more closely at this most painful form of arthritis.

The "crystals" of gout are just that. They are tiny formations of mineral crystals which fill the joint space, causing pain, swelling, and intense irritation. They are caused by an excess of uric acid in the body's fluid composition, which can be produced by a variety of factors. Overeating and drinking is one. So, too, is a genetically determined family disposition toward elevated uric acid production.

Gout can sometimes be difficult to identify. Some years ago, a farmer friend in South Africa hobbled into a neighboring farmhouse saying that he had ". . . a piece of wood in his toe." It had been giving him pain for some time, and he wanted me to remove it. Well, a quick examination revealed nothing so I sent him to the hospital, where he was admitted for surgery to remove the "piece of wood." He was prepared for the operation and was just about to be wheeled into the operating room when a nurse came along with the results of his serum uric acid test. The level was so high that the diagnosis was changed from a wayward splinter to crystal arthritis. He was treated accordingly, but in the nick of time!

The joint tissue's natural attempt to get rid of these crystals is what causes the pain through the process of inflammation. Initially there may be no symptoms, however. Uric acid levels might rise, say, in the bloodstream of pubescent boys or menopausal women without leading to crystal formation. Then, after a particularly rich meal, an attack may occur, most often around the base of the big toe—a form of gout known as podagra. It can strike initially early in the morning, when the toe joint feels so tender, swollen, and sensitive to the touch that the sufferer might for a moment think he had unknowingly broken it the night before.

Other precipitating factors for gout can be the use of diuretics—drugs prescribed to rid excess water from the body in conditions such as heart failure and high blood pressure. These diuretics are known to bring on attacks, as are short stays at health farms where one spends a lot of money for the privilege of being graciously starved of food. Starvation diets elevate uric acid levels in the blood. So losing weight in too drastic a fashion can have adverse consequences for the health of gout joints, not to mention your bank balance. On the other hand, there is no doubt that keeping a check on your weight, avoiding foods high in uric acid (kidney, meat extracts, sardines, heavy beers, port, and strong red wines are among the common culprits), and generally trying to avoid eating and drinking binges will help prevent gout. If you know that your father or his father was a sufferer, these preventive measures make a lot of sense. Would that I had been able to ward off my rheumatoid arthritis with this kind of regime, as I have never been indulgent so far as food is concerned. If you are, you may have to change your habits.

Do not, by the way, think of gout as only attacking the foot. The knee, ankle, shoulder, wrist, and elbow may all be affected, usually only one joint at a time. And do not think of it as one of those millstone-type afflictions that must always remain with you. Prompt diagnosis of your lifestyle (which I will discuss later) will in most cases lead to excellent recovery. The disease of lords and the lord of diseases, for all its long history, can be humbled with modern medicine.

In diagnosing gout an important measurement of course is the level of uric acid in the bloodstream, and there is a test for this. Rheumatologists also look at urine specimens to see how rapidly a sufferer is excreting uric acid, because gout may derive not only from overproduction of uric acid but from a failure to get rid of normal levels. The joint fluid is also examined under the microscope, where it is possible to see quite clearly the unwanted crystal formations when other symptoms have become quite acute.

OTHER FORMS OF ARTHRITIS

My final category of arthritic problems is a big one, including as it does muscle tears, sprains, and general aches and pains, so I will deal only briefly with the various joint and rheumatic conditions included in it. Often the symptoms of some of these complaints are so similar they can easily be confused by doctors. For example, there is a disease called *polymyalgia rheumatica* that affects the hips and shoulders of men and women over about the age of fifty. Now, this is the age at which osteoarthrosis might become a problem, so one's first thought might be to assume that the stiffness and pain do indeed derive from OA. In fact, blood tests show a rise in sedimentation rate which acts as a pointer to polymyalgia rheumatica.

Many joint problems derive from muscle inflammation. Polymyalgia is one. So, too, is *polymyositis*, a condition (see diagram) in which muscle fibers are damaged by the presence of inflammatory cells in regions near the joint. Diagnosis in this case involves investigating levels of biochemical substances called enzymes in the muscle fibers, together with one or two other specialized tests on nerve and muscle functions.

Then there is the group of ailments produced by injury or inflammation such as *bursitis*, seen in such conditions as "housemaid's knee," where the lubricating tissues of the joint—the bursae—become inflamed. The effects are quite localized, often after injury to the painful, swollen area.

We can also include here the general aches and pains of *fibrositis*, which are real enough to the sufferer but frustratingly invisible in laboratory tests. I will be returning to all these problems and more later in the book when we look at available treatments. There is, though, one last form of arthritis that I want to mention here. It is, like RA, a form of synovitis in that it is inflammation of the membranes lining the joint. And, like RA, it is sometimes described as a collagen (or connective tissue) disease. It is also known to be an autoimmune disease—one of those curious disorders in which the body's immune system, instead of confining its activities to defending against infection, declares war on itself. Beyond that, though, the disease—*systemic lupus erythematosus*—is poorly understood. The name *lupus* literally means "wolf," a graphic reminder that sufferers develop a red rash (erythema) across the nose and cheeks that makes the features vaguely wolflike in appearance.

Lupus sufferers vary a good deal. Some barely notice their joint problems. Others are seriously affected by them. The susceptible areas are practically identical with those of RA: knuckles, wrists, sometimes hips and other joints; but in general the effects are less severe. X-rays show few if any abnormalities, as there is hardly ever any erosion of the bone

Muscle inflammation: inflammation among muscle fibers

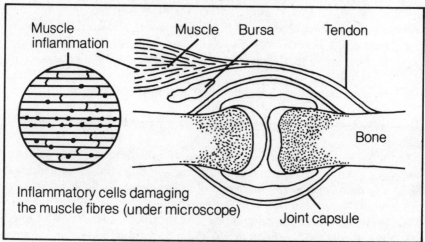

such as you may get with RA. What does happen, though, is one or other of the symptoms: skin rashes and sores, for example, and often kidney troubles such as nephritis. Diagnostic tests for lupus involve checking for antibodies in the blood, which is more revealing than x-rays since there is usually no deformity to be seen.

In general terms, although lupus can be a serious disease—even life threatening in its most extreme form—the prospects for sufferers are good, aided by today's powerful drugs and some changes in lifestyle. More of therapies later. Let us now get back to my rheumatoid arthritis, and how I began to adjust to the role of patient after a lifetime's work as a doctor. It was not easy.

TREATMENT WITH DRUGS   3

Whenever I tell people about my having arthritis, they often look at me in an oddly skeptical way, as if to say, "Oh yes, but you're a doctor. It's all right for you. You know all the drugs and fancy treatments available and can get all sorts of privileges," et cetera, et cetera. They are wrong. Of course as a doctor I know more about joint disease than an untrained person. But there the "privilege" ends. When my arthritis was diagnosed, I felt as depressed and anxious as anyone would in the same position. I was not immune to those slightly irrational fears and feelings we all get in the face of illness, whether our own or that of someone close to us. Nor did I have total, expert knowledge of all the treatment options open to me. If I had, surely I would have been entitled to put "rheumatologist" as well as "cardiologist" on my curriculum vitae.

No, the truth was that, quite aside from my apprehensions about the sort of life rheumatoid arthritis would allow me to lead, I felt, medically speaking, naked. I needed to be told all about the therapies I might have recourse to, immediately and in the future, should the disease remain with me (which seemed to my doctor highly likely) and get worse (which could not be ruled out).

I did what you should do in similar circumstances. I asked questions of my doctor, as many as came into my head during that first diagnostic visit, and on subsequent visits everything that had occurred to me in the meantime. Having an averagely good memory, and no better, I got into the habit of writing down points I wanted to raise. I also read what I could on the subject, confining myself initially to the "respectable" end of the medical literature such as I found in the university libraries, then later venturing into more popular accounts of RA and its treatment. Before long a picture of where I would have to go next began to emerge.

The first thing to hit me was that I need not be a *passive* sufferer, believing and expecting that there was nothing I could do myself to alleviate the pains in my feet and hands. Rheumatoid arthritis, like other forms of arthritis, is not curable, in that there is no course of treatment which will eliminate the disease completely and can therefore be dispensed with once the condition appears to have cleared up. There is, I knew full well, no magical tablet or injection that would act to eradicate my RA in the same way that an antibiotic such as penicillin will comprehensively scourge the body of an infectious bacterium. RA is not like pneumonia. However, the fact that there is no once-and-for-all cure does not mean that RA sufferers should be unduly submissive about their complaint. They need the expert help and support of doctors, of course, in their regular need to take drugs and in choosing the right medication in the first place.

At the same time I discovered both at first and second hand that the sufferer can do something for himself—that treatment, like charity, begins at home. How you live your life, what demands you place on yourself, how you pitch your ambitions and expectations, what you eat and how you work—all these things can play a part in promoting attacks or suppressing them. Later I will be exploring those avenues with you in some detail.

Initially, though, I was very much in my doctor's hands. He had, as I said earlier, given me a ray of hope by saying (rightly or wrongly) that he did not expect me to be crippled by RA. Whether or not his predictions were to prove accurate, it was for me a good start in my new role as patient. Of course, some doctors are better psychologists than others. Mine was a good one. On this point of medical psychology I was always amazed at the approach to disease of some of the surgeons in the United States where I worked. For example, a surgeon would come and say to a man, "You've got cancer of the stomach"—such a direct declaration of hopelessness. Really it's a death sentence. I wouldn't have done it quite that way. My views are so strong that I incorporated them in my book *Good Life/Good Death* (Englewood Cliffs, N.J.: Prentice-Hall, 1980), a discussion about whether terminal patients should be informed or not, or how much they should know. Once I talked to a group of students in Philadelphia about this subject. I said to them that one cannot be too hopelessly brutal. The majority of the students disagreed with me and said that they would want to know if they were going to die. My view is that they were a minority. When there's a little hope and there's a certain quality of life, a person can live quite comfortably until they realize they are seriously ill. If you tell someone that he has a terminal disease, immediately hope is destroyed and the quality of life deteriorates. The interesting thing is there were five or six black students in the class, and they all said they didn't want to know. One cannot make a general rule on this.

Some doctors are much more careful about how they manage the subject, and they don't pronounce a death sentence straightaway. Like this doctor who saw me the first time. I think it could have destroyed me if he had said, "You have got rheumatoid arthritis. I don't know what is going to happen to you, but you may get completely crippled." In some ways having RA was even more alarming to me as a surgeon because it is a condition that cannot be treated quickly. The difference between a surgeon and a physician is that a surgeon can usually see quick results, and that determines how he is motivated and the way he functions. A guy comes to you with a pain in his side and you diagnose acute appendicitis. Three days later he leaves the hospital without acute appendicitis. But when somebody comes to you with diabetes, you never cure the diabetes; you treat the patient with insulin. The same is true for arthritis. So for me to have an incurable disease like RA was a terrible blow because I wanted to get better. I wanted to be fit.

Translating that feeling in everyday practice for the arthritis sufferer means learning about the drugs available for helping you to cope with various manifestations of the disease, or rather group of diseases. You need to understand not only what these drugs do but a little about how they work, because not all act in the same way. Some act, albeit powerfully, only at the level of symptoms, by reducing pain, for example. Others are designed to work at a deeper level, to block the pain-producing process itself, or, as Dr. Alan Hill writes in a publication for the Arthritis and Rheumatism Council, "We can picture these as being able at times to damp the fire down so completely that it may seem to be extinguished." Even with this second group we are still not really talking about a *cure* as such, for, in Dr. Hill's words, "a smouldering core must remain since it bursts back into flame when treatment is stopped—though usually not at once."

We can in fact divide the drugs for treating arthritis into three rather than two categories:

- analgesics (painkillers)
- anti-inflammatory agents
- antirheumatoid drugs

At the end of this chapter I have put all these types of drugs together in a chart for quick reference. First, though, we should look in detail at how these substances act and when they are most appropriate.

ANALGESICS

Pain is an important signal sent by the body and processed in the brain, indicating that something is amiss. For me and I imagine most other arthritis sufferers, the control or at least relief of pain is usually what is most needed most quickly during an attack. Pain can be dulled by highly potent substances such as morphine, but this dangerously addictive drug is clearly of no value for those of us who keep getting painful episodes daily. What we require are preparations such as *acetaminophen,* which belongs to the chemical group known as the aniline derivatives: nonaddictive, fairly fast-acting, freely available, and having hardly any side effects if taken strictly according to the prescribed dosages. Acetaminophen is also a suitable alternative to that other widely used analgesic, aspirin. As we shall see in a moment, aspirin has certain advantages for RA sufferers, but not everyone reacts well to it. It can, for example, produce stomach irritations and upsets.

Acetaminophen has become increasingly popular in recent years, probably being recommended by doctors more often than aspirin, which for a long time was the favorite. However, a word of warning. By all means use this fairly mild, inexpensive analgesic, but never become too cavalier about swallowing a couple of pills whenever you feel a twinge coming on. Acetaminophen overdosing is highly dangerous. It can cause kidney and liver damage and can poison the body, causing anemia and cyanosis (blueness of the lips and skin). If you have anemia or problems of any kind in heart, lung, kidney, or liver function, daily acetaminophen is not to be recommended. Discuss this with your doctor.

Aspirin (acetylsalicylic acid) is present in many compounds and is widely used in treating various forms of arthritis. It can be swallowed in tablet form or dissolved in water. Not only is it a mild analgesic, but it also has an anti-inflammatory action, which is why many physicians understandably tend to use it as a front-line treatment for people with swollen joints.

Much has been written in the popular and medical literature in the last decade or so about the adverse reactions produced by repeated doses of the salicylates, as these compounds are sometimes called. Chief among these are nausea and vomiting, as well as bleeding of the stomach lining. Care should therefore be taken if you need analgesia and anti-inflammatory properties from drugs on a regular basis. Never take aspirin on an empty stomach or if you have a peptic ulcer. Cease taking aspirin if you notice any of the symptoms of "salicylism," which is produced by overdosing: deafness, ringing in the ears, headaches, or nausea. If you have a weak heart, aspirin can be dangerous, as it increases the work of the heart. Doctors think twice about prescribing it to the elderly, the run-down, or women who have heavy menstrual periods because aspirin's effects on the stomach have been implicated in anemia.

That said, aspirin remains a good standby. Proof of its popularity can be judged by the calculation that in the United States alone, 15,000 tons of aspirin are manufactured and swallowed every year. So, reports of gastrointestinal upsets, skin complaints, kidney damage notwithstanding, it remains a valuable drug. Had it just been developed, aspirin might have been classified with the group of substances known as nonsteroidal anti-inflammatory drugs (NSAIDs for short), of which there are nowadays about thirty or forty available for controlling rheumatoid symptoms, often at the expense of aspirin because they have fewer side effects on the stomach lining.

Other drugs in the analgesic group are *phenacetin*, which is no longer recommended because it seems as if it causes kidney damage, and *acetanilid*, a more toxic form of phenacetin which should be avoided.

Remember that whether you use acetaminophen, aspirin, or any other of the analgesics discussed in this chapter, they are painkillers, attacking just a symptom. Pain, ironically, is a necessary evil, alerting us to an underlying medical abnormality that needs attention. It is a warning light. Thus it should not be masked or dulled for too long, for if the warning light is obscured, it cannot continue to act as an indicator to hidden trouble. And, though substances such as acetaminophen are not addictive, it is possible for the body to adjust to them, building up a tolerance, so that one needs increasingly higher doses to get any appreciable effects. High doses can produce unwanted side effects. See further comments about painkillers in Chapter 6.

NONSTEROIDAL ANTI-INFLAMMATORY DRUGS (*NSAIDs*)

Phenylbutazone, sometimes familiarly referred to as "bute," is marketed under a variety of trade names, and, as with any other pharmaceutical preparation, you may have to swap and change, trying out several before finding one that produces the best effects.

Bute has been shown to reduce inflammation in RA, gout, and ankylosing spondylitis. Indeed, for some people it appears to be the only effective preparation for these last two conditions. Unfortunately, however, bute can cause depression of bone marrow activity, producing a drop in the number of white bone cells, a potentially fatal condition which necessitates a bone marrow transplant. Without wanting to sound alarmist, I should point out that there does seem to be evidence that bute—a relatively inexpensive drug—has probably been used by doctors to treat cases where another, less hazardous agent would have been preferable. One British expert told the London *Sunday Times* (15 May 1983) that in ninety-nine cases out of one hundred where bute is prescribed, some other drug would have done just as well. That same article in the *Sunday Times* told the horrifying story of a biochemist who strained her back at work and was prescribed bute by her general practitioner. A few days later she had vaginal irritation, sore throat, and shortly afterward blisters in her mouth. Her reaction was so severe that she had to be hospitalized for six weeks.

Phenybutazone, then, needs to be prescribed with fine clinical judg-ment and taken with extreme caution. It should be obvious to you in a week or so if bute is going to be of benefit. If there is any hint of nausea, stomach upset, weight loss, shortness of breath, or any other side effect such as rashes or sore throat, stop taking the drug and discuss it and your symptoms immediately with your doctor. Do not begin to take it if you have peptic ulcers, high blood pressure, or malfunction of the heart, kid-ney, or liver. The same restrictions and hazards apply to a derivative of bute, *oxyphenbutazone*.

Indomethacin is another NSAID with effects similar to those of aspirin: reduction of inflammation and mild pain relief. RA sufferers benefit from this drug, as do people with gout, attachment arthritis, and sometimes cartilage degeneration. It is sometimes prescribed for systemic lupus.

Indomethacin can have side effects, most commonly headaches and diz-ziness, which usually disappear if the dose is reduced. Other adverse re-actions which are *not* related to the dose taken are loss of appetite, diar-rhea, nausea, vomiting, and dyspepsia. There may also be blood disorders, rashes, and fluid retention. If you have a liver or kidney con-dition, are pregnant, or suffer from peptic ulcers, indomethacin is not for you.

Make sure not to take this drug on an empty stomach, because it can cause internal bleeding. For a time, working long and irregular hours, I used to take indomethacin without thinking carefully about eating before-hand. One day in the bathroom I noticed that my stool was black. Now, the day before I had eaten licorice, so I thought that this was the reason. But the black stools persisted until I began to make a connection between the tablets I was taking and the careless manner of my taking them. I had bled quite badly—a situation I quickly remedied. It was a vivid way to learn caution in drug usage.

Ibuprofen has roughly the same action as indomethacin and can pro-duce similar side effects. Other similar NSAIDs are *fenoprofen* and *na-proxen*.

Tolmetin is an anti-inflammatory drug with some slight analgesic actions which can be used to advantage by a range of arthritis sufferers. I have taken it with benefit for my RA. When I do, I take care and follow the prescribed dosage. Otherwise there is a tendency toward heartburn, in-digestion, and nausea.

Sulindac can also produce gastrointestinal side effects. Sometimes people taking this NSAID report ringing in the ears, headaches, and rashes. A few have had bleeding from the stomach. Again, the pros and cons of this drug should become apparent to anyone taking it for a week or so.

These, then, are some of the popular nonsteroidal anti-inflammatory drugs. But why "nonsteroidal"? Well, this term is, logically enough, to distinguish them from a class of drugs known as the steroids or more properly the corticosteroids, for which I personally have enormous reason to be grateful.

CORTICOSTEROIDS

These compounds were introduced with considerable fanfare in the 1950s, widely hailed as "miracle medicines" and "wonder drugs" by enthusiastic doctors and their patients. They had been developed by three researchers—Edward C. Kendall, Tadeus Reichstein, and Philip S. Hench—who in 1950 shared a Nobel Prize for showing that these hormones would suppress symptoms of inflammation and allergy. Now, more than once it has been suggested to me that I have earned a Nobel Prize for being the world's first heart transplant surgeon. But I have always found that idea ridiculous. Mine was undeniably an achievement. It needed certain skills and techniques. I had to enthuse, inspire even, and lead a large team of people, each with a specialized role to play. I had to do the actual surgery. But when I think of the intellectual and imaginative power of people like Kendall, Reichstein, and Hench, I see my own work in perspective. I appreciate that if there are to be such institutions as medical prizes, then the highest honors should go to people who advance mankind solely by the power of thought.

Anyway, back to the corticosteroids. These substances were rapidly seized on by rheumatologists for their instant effects on inflammation, but soon it began to emerge that there were disadvantages to outweigh the benefits. Dr. Peter Wingate, in the *Penguin Medical Encyclopedia*, sums up the dilemma they provoked: "Inflammation has unpleasant and sometimes dangerous effects, but it is fundamentally a defensive reaction. To suppress it indiscriminately is like abolishing the fire brigade to stop it from breaking windows and doors." In other words, corticosteroids—in particular, *cortisone*—began to produce in patients other symptoms that were less desirable than the inflammation the drug had suppressed. It can lead to thinning of the bones, stomach troubles, high blood pressure, skin disorders, and in some people a prominent and distressing swelling of the face and body.

On the other hand, I can remember times when, in total agony from joint pains, a steroid injection has relieved the pain in a miraculous way. I am not the only person to feel like this. Here is the experience of Maureen Mason, an arthritis sufferer who took part in a BBC World Service broadcast, "Assignment—Arthritis" (Oct. 22, 1980):

> I felt unwell, really quite unwell, like having to sit down to wash up and that sort of thing, and I was in a lot of pain—crying even sometimes and feeling very depressed because I thought, well, if it goes on like this, you

know, I'd become so stiff and with a lot of pain so quickly in comparison, I mean it wasn't as much or anything like what other people put up with, but rather quickly, I thought if it's going to go on like this, you know, in no time at all I'm going to be, you know, completely bedridden.

I went into hospital almost as soon as I saw the rheumatologist. As soon as the blood tests had come through he advised me to go into hospital for complete rest and also for injections into the joints, so I was in hospital for ten days absolutely as a bed patient. I was put on drugs of course, and also with these injections, which helped enormously, I mean, they were just almost miraculous. Certainly it was something that really did take the pain away in a very short time indeed, and the effects lasted for quite a while after you'd had them. Perhaps I'm wrong in saying I had daily ones, but he certainly would come along with all the kit and would give me the injections in the fingers and in the knees.

The drug used in Maureen's case was in fact cortisone.

Now, steroids have an added significance for me as a transplant expert because they act not only on inflammation but on the immune system—they suppress the body's natural tendency to reject foreign tissue, including, of course, another person's heart. Here, too, there are problems. To stop rejection I have to administer large doses, which means that my patient is, for a time, unprotected from disease and infections. He or she could succumb to a bacterium, while the new heart is working perfectly. So even as I began to take cortisone for my own arthritis, I was aware that using those powerful drugs was an exercise in risk-benefit analysis. I knew that for all the relief they would afford me, I had to face possible consequences in other ways. An American rheumatologist once told me that once you take steroid substances you have "a tiger by the tail"! Being anabolic agents, these drugs tend to lead to muscle wastage. Did I really want to take a drug to prevent arthritis from incapacitating me when that same substance was likely to do exactly the same thing in another way? Well, all I can say is that with your doctor's help this is something you have to try to work out for yourself.

Recently I was invited on board a friend's boat off the Greek island of Kos when traveling on a lecture tour of Europe. At the time my steroids were with most of my luggage on a cruise liner in the harbor, so I stayed the night with my friend without them. Next morning they virtually had to carry me off that ship because my joints were so stiff and sore. I went back to my cabin on the liner and took fifteen milligrams of steroids by mouth and went to sleep. About six hours later I woke up with no pain at all. Given a drug that does that to me, it is very difficult for me in all honesty to be too reticent about the benefits of corticosteroids. Not only do they dampen swelling in the joints but they also generally affect the whole body, giving a sense of well-being—almost a "high." They really do work but they must, repeat *must,* be taken with caution. My doctor advises me never to take them for long stretches at a time because they affect the body's fundamental metabolism. He puts me on low-dose treatments if he can, and avoids the drugs altogether if possible.

If I have made the use of corticosteroids sound a bit enigmatic, that is precisely what it is. Dr. Wingate believes that the decision whether or not to prescribe them is "among the most difficult in current medical practice. A patient with RA who has once experienced the immediate improvement that corticosteroids can bring may take a lot of persuading that on balance her particular case is better treated without them." I agree wholeheartedly.

I tend to take them by mouth, by the way, but they can be administered also by injection into the painful area. Sometimes it is possible to stimulate the body into generating more of its own hormone production by injecting a special cortical stimulating hormone called ACTH.

Anti-arthritis steroids are marketed under a variety of brand names (see chart on page 58–60), but the compound most usually given in tablet form is *prednisone* (and *prednisolone*). Sometimes this drug will produce a somewhat paradoxical effect in people who reduce their dose. They get a condition known as steroid fibrositis, in which the joints are more stiff and painful for a week or so. Not unnaturally, this is often instantly thought of as an ominous sign that the original arthritic condition is returning. So if such a phenomenon occurs to you, do not leap to the obvious conclusion but talk immediately to your doctor—without stepping up the dose of prednisone in the meantime.

Watch out for an increase in weight. Prednisone tends to sharpen the appetite as well as to encourage the body to retain more fluid. No one with arthritis—or without it, for that matter—can afford to carry excess baggage by way of body fat.

ANTIMALARIAL DRUGS

Before we leave the anti-inflammatory drugs, steroidal or nonsteroidal, there is another group of substances which has been of some help to me and a number of other sufferers, even though their mode of action in combating RA is still slightly mysterious. The compounds are in the *chloroquine* family, which were originally developed for treating malaria. They certainly reduce swelling in synovitis and reduce the red skin problems in lupus and have few side effects. That said, there is a remote possibility of visual disorders occurring; blindness even can result in some people. Regular eye tests are required, especially for red vision, which is the first to become affected. Again, then, proceed with caution. Chloroquine (and hydroxychloroquine) can be used in association with an analgesic like aspirin, which means that you can, under doctor's orders, keep a regulatory check on dosage.

ANTIRHEUMATOID DRUGS

The antirheumatoid drugs are substances which act in some way to alter the very disease process itself, rather than alleviate its symptoms. These are sometimes called drugs to induce remissions. Perhaps the most evocative compound in this group is the most precious of metals, *gold*, a substance which has fascinated mankind in general for many hundreds of years and doctors in particular for the past three decades. Funnily enough, the use of gold salts for treating RA came about by a happy accident. Some doctors thought, mistakenly, that RA was caused by the tubercle bacillus, the organism responsible for tuberculosis. They thought of RA, if you like, as a "tuberculosis of the joints." Now, gold used to be prescribed for treating tuberculosis—not, I should stress, with much success—so it seemed reasonable enough at least to give it a try for arthritis. To the great delight of doctors and patients, gold showed itself to be dramatically effective initially, though then, as now, it was not clear why it works as well as it does. Then, as with cortisone, side effects of a serious nature began to be noticed, so for a time gold—the eternally valuable commodity—practically went out of therapeutic circulation. In more recent years it has made something of a comeback, primarily because doctors have been more careful in using smaller amounts and have followed up gold injections with blood and urine tests to monitor any unwelcome side effects, as well as the benefits.

The side effects of gold only really show up when a considerable amount has been administered, because these salts circulate very slowly in the body's tissues. When they do, they can take a variety of forms: skin complaints, kidney and blood disorders, and bone marrow disorders are the most important, but mouth ulcers, nausea, sometimes mild hepatitis can also occur. It has been estimated that even with current techniques, one in four people being treated with gold will have to come off it as a result of side effects. On the other hand, seven out of ten patients show improvements, sometimes substantial.

Unlike some of the other drugs I have been discussing, gold takes time to show how beneficial it can be. So be patient. You may have to wait as much as a couple of months or more before you recognize any alleviation in your symptoms.

The other main category of antirheumatoids is the *penicillamines*, which are made as a by-product of the manufacture of the best known of all antibiotics, penicillin. These drugs have side effects similar to those produced by gold, and they also take months to act on your symptoms. So, as with gold, doctors like to monitor carefully the blood and urine of patients taking penicillamine to check on progress and any adverse effects. Since I travel so much, I find it difficult to take gold or penicillamines regularly. One needs to be monitored by a doctor carefully, so these drugs are not for people who lead an irregularly patterned life.

These, then, are the main classes of drugs you are likely to meet with as an arthritis sufferer. I have deliberately not mentioned each and every type of drug that *could* be used, because any that I have not mentioned will require even closer discussion with your doctor before deciding on their use. Doctors vary as well. Some, for example, may prefer to recommend *codeine* for pain relief, even though this is potentially addictive, can cause several complications, and is frowned on by other rheumatologists. Or your doctor may ask you whether you want to try an immunosuppressant drug to try to combat an arthritic condition that seems auto-immune in origin. These drugs can be powerful and hazardous and need very careful administration and monitoring. Then there are newly developed experimental drugs or drugs with very specific actions (for combating, say, uric acid overproduction in gout), all of which have features that merit attention and discussion. My advice is to ask as many questions as you can: about length of time you will need to take the tablets offered, how they act, what their side effects are, what their dangers and their potential benefits are. If the drug is newly developed, ask your doctor whether it genuinely offers something that other compounds already tried and tested on the market cannot provide. Play for safety, not spectacular overnight results. There are no miracles in medicine. Superb, marvelous treatments, but no miracles.

DRUGS FOR TREATING ARTHRITIS

NAME OF DRUG	USES	POSSIBLE SIDE EFFECTS
Analgesics		
acetylsalicylic acid (aspirin)	Pain relief, especially for cartilage degeneration, local conditions; anti-inflammatory in RA, synovitis generally, and attachment arthritis such as ankylosing spondylitis	Nausea, vomiting, headaches, allergic reactions, ulcers, breathing disorders, anemia
acetaminophen (Tylenol)	Mild, temporary pain relief	Liver and kidney damage in overdose, cyanosis, anemia
phenacetin	Mild, temporary pain relief	Liver and kidney damage in overdose, cyanosis, anemia
propoxyphene (Darvon)	Mild pain relief in short term	Mental dullness, dizziness, headache, rashes, stomach upset
codeine	Moderate pain relief, but prescribed comparatively rarely because of both addictive properties and side effects	Constipation, nausea, drowsiness
Nonsteroidal Anti-Inflammatory Drugs (NSAIDs)		
phenylbutazone (Azolid, Butazolidin)	Gout, synovitis, attachment arthritis, local conditions	Anemia, stomach upset, nausea, heartburn, fluid retention, ulcers, blurred vision, bone marrow depression
oxyphenbutazone (Oxalid, Tandearil)	Gout, synovitis, attachment arthritis, local conditions	Anemia, stomach upset, nausea, heartburn, fluid retention, ulcers, blurred vision
indomethacin (Indocin)	Gout, synovitis, attachment arthritis, local conditions	Headache, dizziness, nausea, stomach upset, heartburn
ibuprofen (Motrin)	Attachment arthritis, synovitis, local conditions	Headache, dizziness, nausea, stomach upset, heartburn, sometimes fever, stiff neck with lupus patients

fenoprofen (Nalfon)	Attachment arthritis, synovitis, local conditions, gout	Stomach upset, nausea, fluid retention occasionally
naproxen (Naprosyn)	Attachment arthritis, synovitis, local conditions, gout	Stomach upset, nausea, fluid retention occasionally
tolmetin (Tolectin)	Synovitis, attachment arthritis, gout, some local conditions	Stomach upset, nausea, fluid retention occasionally
sulindac (Clinoril)	Synovitis, attachment arthritis, gout, some local conditions	Stomach upset, nausea, fluid retention occasionally, ringing in the ears, itching, and nervous disorders

Corticosteroids

prednisone, prednisolone (Delta-Cortef, Deltasone, Orasone, Meticorten)	Mainly reduces inflammation in muscles and connective tissue diseases, also RA and other forms of synovitis	Many and varied, according to the regime prescribed, including ulcers, skin problems, depression, overweight, bruising, facial hair growth, softening of bones, stretch marks on skin, cataracts
triamcinolone hexacetonide and others (steroid injections marketed under a variety of trade names)	Reduces inflammation of noninfectious kind	Relatively few, but bone damage can occur after series of injections
ACTH (injections marketed under a variety of trade names)	Reduces inflammation	Same as for prednisone

Antirheumatoid Drugs

gold salts (Myochrysine)	Reduces inflammation in synovitis such as RA	Skin problems, blood disorders, kidneys, ulcers, nausea, hepatitis (mild)
penicillamine (Cuprimine)	Synovitis	As above, plus delayed healing of cuts

Antigout Compounds

colchicine	Relieves gout attacks and prevents arthritis	Diarrhea, stomach ache
probenecid (Benemid)	Reduces blood uric acid levels in acute gout patients	Negligible
allopurinol (Lopurin, Zyloprim)	Reduces uric acid levels in blood and urine	Minimal, but possibly skin rashes, stomach upset

DRUGS FOR TREATING ARTHRITIS (*Continued*)

NAME OF DRUG	USES	POSSIBLE SIDE EFFECTS
Immunosuppressants		
cyclophosphamide (Cytoxan)	Lupus, RA and a few other arthritic conditions where there is need to shut down immune system	Infections, hair loss, bladder problems, possibility of cancer after long-term use
chlorambucil (Leukeran)	Same as above	Same as above, without bladder problems
azathioprine (Imuran) 6-mercaptopurine (Purinethol) }	Lupus, RA in severe forms, and some other serious conditions requiring immunosuppression	Infections, stomach upset, possibility of cancer
methotrexate	Immunosuppression	Same as above
Tranquilizers		
diazepam (Valium) chlordiazepoxide (Librium) }	Promotes cheerfulness and aid sleep	Various: drowsiness, fatigue, sometimes rashes, constipation, incontinence, and trembling

KEYS TO SELF-MANAGEMENT 4

For all the drugs already available and currently being tested, most forms of arthritis, including rheumatoid arthritis, are not treatable so much as manageable. This idea of managing an illness as opposed to treating it comprehensively or curing it outright was impressed upon me right from the start. I would, the rheumatologists told me, have to make concessions in life, have to learn to listen to the signals coming to me from my body, have to modify my way of living and working to try to accommodate myself to the RA.

Frankly, I found this impossible in the early days. On the one hand, I was aware of the "signals," in the form of pain, but knew that drugs really did nothing more than make life as bearable as possible. I know all the drugs because I have used virtually all of the anti-inflammatory agents that calm down the pain and the others which give remission, such as gold, penicillimine, and chloroquine. On the other hand, try as I might, I could not shrug off that repeated feeling of having been cheated by fate. You have, the doctor said (as I have done myself to patients), got to accept the facts of your case—a slowly progressing but inescapable disease. But for some people it is easier to accept than for others. For me it has always been very difficult. I felt it was the worst thing that could have happened to me because of my tremendous drive and ambition and pride. I could never be philosophical and thank God that I only had arthritis and not something more incapacitating.

I kept on saying to God, "Why did I have to get arthritis? Where have I sinned that I have come to the wretched state that I am now in today? If I am being punished, what am I being punished for?" And so on and so forth. Added to this mish-mash of emotions was another element that I want to admit to: the feeling not only of incapacity or restriction but stigma. Arthritis so far as I am concerned was, although not life-threatening, one of the worst afflictions that could have entered my life because it is so visible.

61

The worst diseases, I feel, are those where people around you see you have got it. If you have a hole in the heart, nobody is aware of it. So it's not as bad as having a faceful of acne that other people can see. Those are perhaps the worst diseases to have—unsightly dermatological conditions, diseases that greatly reduce the quality of life. That is why I see nothing wrong with having face lifts and bags under the eyes removed surgically and things like that. I would have had myself done if I felt my quality of life would be improved by it. At my stage now, it is difficult to cover up the fact that I am crippled, and it hurts my pride. I cannot generalize; I must speak only for myself. Some people don't mind it very much, but I do mind it very much. I also mind when my children see that I am struggling. There is something in the way they look at me which I cannot bear. So as far as diseases are concerned, the worst ones for me to have are those where you are not only suffering from it physically but you have the emotional trauma that other people see you have the disease. So while I pray God that I don't get cancer, the tumor itself is not the thing that worries me, it is the slow falling to pieces that accompanies the illness.

Given these feelings, then, I had, to say the least, an uphill struggle not to be overwhelmed by my arthritis. Drugs would kill pain and, in the case of steroid injections, produce remarkable, sometimes seemingly miraculous remissions. When for the first time I developed severe arthritic symptoms in my knee joints, whereas hitherto the pain and swelling had been localized in my hands and feet, steroid injections gave me complete remission. And so far I have had no recurrence worth mentioning. Yet my hands and feet continued to grow worse, with only temporary improvements from tablets or injections. Was this, I asked myself, the best I could hope for? The beginning of the end of my story as a successful doctor, keen sportsman, and most important of all, active husband and father? Was there nothing I could do for myself to improve matters?

Even as I posed the question to myself, I knew the answer. My rheumatologist had made it perfectly plain that there was a lot more to arthritis management than simply acting as a mindless vessel for whatever drugs he chose to give me. There were practical initiatives I could take to meet the disease halfway. The problem really lay in myself, in my own mental attitudes toward what I despairingly insisted on treating as my unique cross that God or fate had forced me to bear. With hindsight I was probably more than a little self-pitying. Then something, or rather two things, happened to change my attitude, to enable me to see myself in quite a different perspective.

The first was that a friend of mine developed cancer of the colon with secondary growth. He was operated on, but he realized that he had secondaries in the liver and therefore he couldn't be cured. But it was fascinating and inspiring to see how much he tried to do in the few months that he lived. I was not in the country when he died, but I believe that when he was in the terminal phase he kept asking the attending physicians to allow him to live just one more day because he still had things that he wanted to achieve. I am not consciously aware that the thought of having limited time to practice surgery really stimulated me to be more enthusiastic or to work harder. However, I am sure that subconsciously this has been a stimulus. So while I never said to myself, "Well, you know you are only going to be able to operate for two or three more years and you will only be able to do this research for a few more years and therefore you must do as much as you can," I think that my friend's death was for me a reminder that whatever life I had left—with or without arthritis—I could continue to extract something from it.

The second event was even more salutary, because it taught me the importance not of what one has "lost" but of what one has left. I saw a child one morning at the Red Cross Hospital who had been admitted with a tragically severe burn in the esophagus, due to mistakenly swallowing some caustic soda. His esophagus was totally constricted so that he couldn't even swallow his own saliva which built up in his mouth. He could chew but not swallow his food, so an arrangement was rigged up whereby it was collected via a tube running from his neck and dropping its contents into a little bag. In all, a wretched condition for any adult let alone a child to suffer. On the day I was there I saw this boy in the ward eating and playing happily with his friends. He chewed his food and it duly fell in the bag on the side of his neck. When he finished he smiled, rose from his chair, saying "Well, I enjoyed that," and left the table, whereupon he went into a small room off the ward where nurses emptied the bag and fed him properly through a tube into the stomach. Although having breakfast with his friends provided no nourishment for the body, it did much for the happiness and personality of that remarkable little boy. He wanted to be a normal, sociable individual and he managed to be so by making, it seemed to me, use of what he had left: the ability to communicate.

From that day I began to concentrate less on what I had lost and more on what was left and to use, exploit, develop, and maintain it to the full.

My first major step along the admittedly arduous path to self-management was a matter of improving my mental attitude. I have never been one to have recourse to tranquilizers or antidepressants when things look bleak, but I might well have done so. RA sufferers often experience many of the classic signs of depression and anxiety; they worry about the future generally and about jobs, income, and family life in particular. They can lose sleep as well as enthusiasm and zest for living, and certainly antidepressant drugs may be useful to get them over these hurdles. But only, I suspect, in the beginning. For a long-term change of attitude you need to find your own solution within yourself. I was lucky in having two courageous examples to inspire me—and as a doctor, of course, I have been privileged to witness many such people who fight on regardless of pain or deprivation. For most arthritis sufferers the best route out of depression—with, as I say, occasional help from antidepressant drugs—is to talk out your worries into a sympathetic ear. It could be a spouse, a relative, a friend, or a professional listener in the shape of a counselor or psychotherapist. Elderly people living alone are certainly at a disadvantage here because their range of social contacts may of necessity be limited. Again, though, if there is no friendly neighbor or acquaintance to act as listener, you may still get help through your doctor in the form of a nurse or social worker, trained not only to listen but to offer experienced advice to dispel those fears. One thing is clear. The more you articulate the things that depress you, the less depressing they become. Conversely, depression and arthritis seem to fuel each other. If you succumb to one, you will aggravate the other. Sitting around worrying about what might or might not happen at some vague time in the future does not help an arthritic condition. And this brings me to my second step in self-management: exercise.

I have always been physically active, a tendency which has stood me in good stead as an arthritic. True, it caused one problem in that I found to my great dismay that as my RA progressed, it robbed me of the chance to play as often as I would like with my young children. They would play with bats and balls, both tennis and cricket, and they would ask me to play with them. I would often try and bat, but every time I attempted to hit the ball, the jarring impact of the ball on the bat would give me tremendous pain in my hands and wrists. Or when I tried to bowl, it was impossible because of the pain in my shoulders. If they asked me to swim with them, I couldn't crawl overhand anymore because of the pain. I could not kick a ball because of the pains in my feet. This was all very frustrating and distressing, the feeling that I was letting them down. But on the other hand, I have never taken what I call the wheelchair option in arthritis. Prolonged inactivity is not for me, if I can help it; I reckon that, so far as mobility of limbs and joints is concerned, it is a question of "Use it or lose it."

Exercise in some form or another is indispensable to health. We are not machines that wear out with constant use. Indeed, the human body will deteriorate more rapidly without exercise than with it. Bone is an unusual substance. The more activity you impose on it, the stronger it becomes. The same is true of the six hundred or so muscles in our bodies. Tendons and ligaments, too, increase in strength in response to exercise, as does the cartilage—the layer of joint gristle—which depends for its nourishment on the compression action produced by the moving joint.

So if you have any joint problems, some form of exercise, consistent with what is comfortable, practicable, and enjoyable, has a number of direct arthritis-related benefits. And if you are bothered by worry and anxiety, there is an added reason to exercise. Doesn't everyone feel more at peace emotionally and intellectually after a pleasant swim or game of tennis than after just sitting around? *Mens sana in corpore sano* (a healthy mind in a healthy body) is not, as it is often caricatured, just the motto of some hearty British public school. It is, to my satisfaction at least, established fact given widespread medical approval.

So exercise is an important item in our anti-arthritis program. The next question in your mind will be: What exercise, how much, and how often?

To take the question of frequency first, you should aim for regularity of activity rather than the occasional sporting binge. Better to walk three miles at a gentle pace every day or spend ten minutes on some morning or evening exercises in a chair than attempt to be the hardest-hitting squash player in the district once a week—with nothing in between.

Next the question of how much exercise is appropriate. Here you should remember that inflammatory conditions such as RA can temporarily get worse after exercise. That means you should balance exercise carefully with rest periods. There seems, incidentally, to be something of a controversy among doctors on this question of rest. Rest, it is true, will reduce inflammation, but its effects on bone, muscle, tendon, and cartilage are just the opposite to those of exercise. So there is clearly a cost-benefit equation to be worked out, and I can think of no better guidelines than those offered by Dr. James F. Fries in his excellent book, *Arthritis: and How to Cope with It* (London: Granada, 1980). He states: "The consensus [among doctors] is that exercise is necessary for all patients with all forms of arthritis. With active synovitis, exercise should be limited [while the active inflammation persists] to levels that do not greatly increase the pain and inflammation." In short, tune in again to the signals from your body. If a particular activity or sport or exercise produces pain, back off and find a gentle alternative or approach the activity more slowly. You will find that you can work up to higher levels of exercise by beginning modestly than you can by trying to start near the top.

I have been talking generally about exercise to cover all sorts of activities from walking (instead of taking the bus) to sports to exercise programs proper. The first category should be always in your mind for general health purposes. Not only will your joints remain more supple longer, but your heart will pump more strongly, your circulation be improved, and your weight will stay down—all desirable bonuses. As for the second, you either like sports or you do not. In my mid-forties it was inconceivable to me that I should give up swimming or horseback riding, both of which I love doing. On the other hand, if you are a town dweller in your fifties or sixties who has not done anything remotely sporty since your school days, it is a different matter. So for you, perhaps the third category of purpose-built exercise programs will be most appropriate. In that case, you will find something to interest you in Chapter 10.

Before we move on to other self-management measures, though, I want to discuss an aspect of arthritis that people frequently, and understand-ably, raise with me. If, they ask, arthritis is a problem limited to one or two joints, why not try a once-and-for-all cure by surgery? Can other sur-geons do for the RA sufferer what I and other transplant doctors have been able to do for people with defective kidneys, corneas, or hearts? In short, for the arthritic, how about spare-parts surgery? Well, I can appreciate why people might ask these questions, and in the next chapter I will try to provide the answers.

SPARE-PARTS OPERATIONS AND
OTHER SURGICAL TREATMENTS

5

Arthritis has been linked to the motor car; although there is a huge variety of types, they are all fundamentally related. Arthritis takes many forms, each producing its own set of problems for the sufferer. Like the cars streaming by on the road outside, each is different, though the basic template—joint trouble—is roughly the same. That said, the comparison has one major limitation. If your car develops a running fault in the region of the crankshaft or the pistons and this cannot be overcome by tightening a few nuts and replacing a gasket or two, you may be able to put the vehicle back on the road in perfect running order overnight simply by replacing the defective parts. It matters not whether they are large or small. You can cure any mechanical fault in an inanimate piece of equipment by spare-parts surgery, engineering style. Or, if it is convenient, you can unfasten the faulty component, mend it at leisure on the workbench, then replace it, good as new. With arthritis, things are simply not like that. It is never a question of automatically replacing an old painful joint with a freely moving artificial one—and for some arthritic conditions the question of surgery never even arises. Nor is the procedure a trivial one, like having a filling put into a tooth cavity. Surgery is often rightly viewed as a last-resort procedure, not unlike open-heart surgery, where all other measures to maintain a patient in good health have failed.

At the same time, for some conditions, such as osteoarthritis, surgery is often the only effective treatment, which is something of a paradox. All the painkillers and anti-inflammatory agents in the world will not halt the progression of OA, any more than two aspirin will slow down tooth decay. So if and when surgery is recommended for a person immobilized by OA, there is invariably some medical algebra to do: the calculation of risk against benefit. A leading bone and joint surgeon, Dr. Michael Freeman of the London Hospital, expresses the issue thus: "You have to weigh against the attraction of being rid of the pain in your hip or your knee the disadvantage of exposing yourselves to the risks and the unpleasantness of surgery."

Many arthritics are, as I said earlier, never even faced with this choice (and, in some cases, dilemma) because surgery is simply not applicable to their problem. Generally speaking, surgery, as you might expect, is most effective in treating localized joint problems. If, like me, you have a condition which originally affected one foot and has moved to both feet, then the hands and fingers, and is likely to progress to the knees and elbows, then surgery may be an impractical solution. I found this a frustrating but necessary realization to come to, having built my career on what you might call "positive surgery"—the use of operations to restore the quality of life to patients who otherwise would have been infirm.

So as a rule (though it is not an inflexible one), surgery is best for local, definable conditions. Then the joint itself may not be very accessible to the surgeon. Or, for some other technical reason, it may not be possible to replace it, or if it is, the spare part may be less than perfect. There are usually other factors entering into the decision. For example, the age of the sufferer could lead a doctor to decide that, on balance, an operation is undesirable. Large joints such as the hip and knee have, so far at least, given the best results in surgical repair or replacement operations. In fact, the prospects here are remarkably cheerful compared to surgery on smaller joints, where sophisticated repair methods do not always lead to the increase in function achieved in larger-scale operations.

For all the restrictions and conditions surrounding surgery, it is arguable that this century's greatest advance in the treatment of arthritis has come in the realm of surgical operations. Hip joint replacement or arthroplasty is carried out about a quarter of a million times a year around the world, with the very high success rate of 85 percent. In Britain alone, according to Professor Verna Wright, a rheumatologist from Leeds University, up to forty thousand people a year gain tremendous relief from hip replacement procedures. Not everyone is uniformly delighted with the new hip, though. Some sufferers, especially the elderly, may have other medical problems, so that while their osteoarthritic hip is "cured" overnight, they are still not 100 percent fit. Some people, according to British psychologist Karen Barton, are disappointed by the results of their operation. It is "successful" in the strictly surgical sense but still does not come up to the patient's expectations. So if you and your doctor are talking along lines that seem to be leading toward a hip replacement operation, try to find out in as much detail as you can (and this is not easy for you or your doctor) precisely what you can expect to gain from it.

Do not be afraid to probe your doctor on this. Patient-doctor communication is, in my view, a much neglected aspect of medical life. It is increasingly being realized by the medical profession that doctors have a

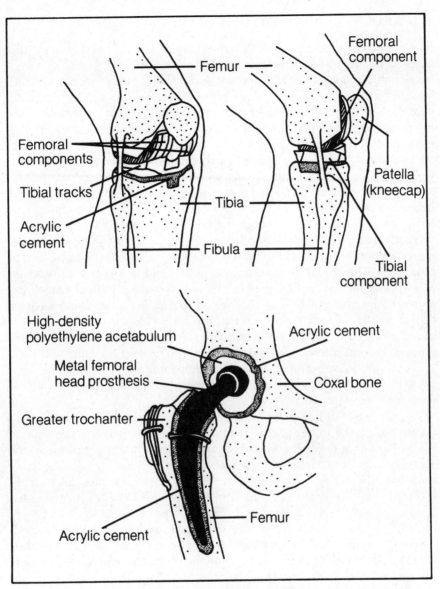

Total hip and total knee replacement. *Top:* two total knee replacement prostheses. In the polycentric type of technique (*left*), there are two femoral and two tibial components. In the Waldius technique (*right*) there are one femoral component and one tibial component. *Bottom:* Charnley's technique and prosthesis for total hip relacement. The arthritic portions of the acetabulum and head of the femur are replaced by a prefabricated joint. The acetabulum is made of a polyethylene substance of high density, and the metallic femoral head is cemented into the femur with acrylic cement. The greater trochanter of the femur is reattached after surgery.

duty to impart knowledge and advice to their patients, as well as to dispense care of a strictly therapeutic kind. More and more emphasis is, I am delighted to say, being placed on "social skills," "personal interaction," "counseling roles," and so on in the training programs of medical students, who should be better equipped than many doctors of my generation were to talk frankly and freely to their charges. Personally I have always felt it important to try to describe before an operation exactly what I intend to do and what I expect to achieve with every patient. There is nothing worse than the person who, having undergone the major and, let us face it, traumatic experience of a big operation, feels that he was tricked into it because it fails to live up to his expectations. Trust is always important—before and after the patient is wheeled into the operating room.

Another attendant problem of surgery—*any* surgery, be it for hip replacement or removal of an ingrown toenail—is that infections can occur, however stringent the precautions taken to avoid them. It does not happen very often, but often enough for the surgeon Sir John Charnley, pioneer of the artificial hip, to have developed a "clean air tent" for joint operations. It is basically an operating theater within a theater, a tent from which air is constantly flowing outward, and carrying with it any potentially dangerous microorganisms that could be floating around.

These, then, are some of the qualifications one would have to make to the otherwise successful procedure of hip replacement. Let us look at how joint replacements actually work.

The hip was the first joint to be replaced, and nowadays these superb operations can be either partial or total. In a partial operation the femoral head (the ball of the ball-and-socket arrangement) or the acetabulum (the socket) can be replaced. A total replacement operation involves installing both ball and socket at the same time. There are various designs of artificial hips available to surgeons to implant, the best known of which is the Charnley prosthesis (see diagram). Earlier types such as the Judet were effective initially but tended to wear badly and had to be removed, whereas a patient today can expect ten to fifteen years' wear, depending on the loads imposed, and current bio-engineering research will certainly extend that usable lifetime in the near future.

There is a lot of intriguing technology in the artificial hip: in the plastics and metals used; in the cements employed to hold them in place; in experiments on alternative materials such as hard-wearing ceramics. Not without justification does Sir John Charnley call the total joint replacement operations "probably the most exciting and rewarding development in orthopaedic surgery in the last twenty years." (ARC Publication)

Suppose that you are to have a hip joint replaced. What would the operation and its aftermath be like for you? Here's a description of the whole process by Michael Freeman, as he related on the BBC's "Assignment—Arthritis" (Oct. 22, 1980):

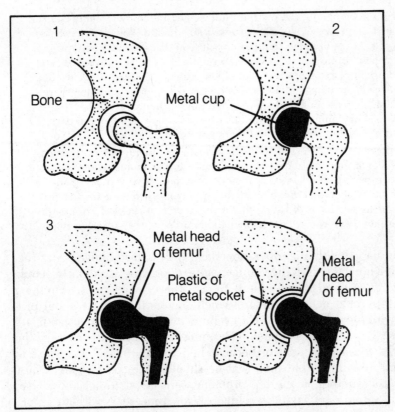

Hip arthroplasties: (1) normal hip; (2) interposition; (3) partial replacement; (4) total replacement

The day of the operation you're pre-medicated—that means you have an injection in your bed and you're a little sleepy; you're then anaesthetized and the surgeon then makes a cut over the hip joint, he removes the diseased bone from the hip joint and he replaces it with a man-made ball and socket (the socket is made from plastic, the ball is typically made of metal) and the two are fixed to the living bone of your skeleton with a cold curing acrylic that moulds itself on the one hand to the implant and on the other hand to the skeleton and then he closes the wound and the anaesthetist arranges that you wake up, and then in something like an hour or two hours later you're coming round and you have not a very wonderful day for the rest of the day. You've got an infusion going in your arm because you can't drink for yourself and you're a bit uncomfortable so you're given injections for that, but by the next day the infusion comes down and typically you see the patient at breakfast time, they're sitting up and starting to have their breakfast and there they are. The next day—that's day 2—some little drains that are put in the leg to take the excess blood that may have leaked around the tissues to take it out of the leg altogether, they're removed and when they're removed the patient can get up out of bed, can put their full weight on their leg, but of course it is a consequence of any major surgery to a joint of this kind that it has the reflex effect of paralysing the muscles, so that although you can put your weight on the leg it's as if you were putting it on a paralysed leg and you therefore have to use sticks or elbow crutches or something, just like a paralysed person would do, otherwise you'd fall down. And then there's a gradual increase in muscle power, and physio-therapy has a part to play there in shortening that period, but we're talking roughly of ten days to go out of hospital with a wound that's got the stitches out, able to go up and down stairs, dressed, able to manage at home with some non-professional support, and a couple of sticks; and at about six weeks starting to progress off sticks or crutches. Now that's a very rough guide, I mean, that shouldn't be thought of by anyone listening to this programme as some sort of law so that if you're still on sticks at two months something extraordinary has happened. (Source: BBC External Services)

It often happens that an operation such as described above is not recommended for arthritis in the younger age groups, whereas elderly people are encouraged to go ahead with it. In fact, there seems to be something of a cutoff point at age fifty, before which doctors think twice about proceeding with hip replacement. They tend to ask the prospective candidate for a prosthesis whether he (or she) is coming for treatment because of the state of the hip as it is now, or because he fears that it will get worse in future and he will be told then that he should have come sooner. They also will ask whether, if the hip problem were never to get any worse, would the sufferer be happy to soldier on for some years without an operation. Usually the answers point to postponing the surgery, unless the state of the hips means a person cannot continue to earn a living.

It is, I should point out, a false idea that better results will come from having a total hip replacement sooner rather than later. Remember, too, that any synthetic spare parts, of metal and plastic, will be subject to wear, and that it is not possible to guarantee that the prosthesis will last as long as you do, especially if you are active at sports or have a physically demanding job. For these reasons, too, total hip replacement—though it is one of the surgical success stories of modern medicine—will on occasion be discouraged among younger people.

With the knee, orthopedic surgeons can also claim considerable success, though not as comprehensively as with the hip. With its ball-and-socket structure, the hip, though a complex piece of natural biological engineering, is easier to reproduce by artificial means because, unlike the knee, it does not have to resist sideways force. Imagine a knee joint built like a hip. The leg bones would hinge freely enough, but they would also splay out sideways, whereas walking and running require that they come into a rigid alignment. Again ingenuity has not been spared to find suit-

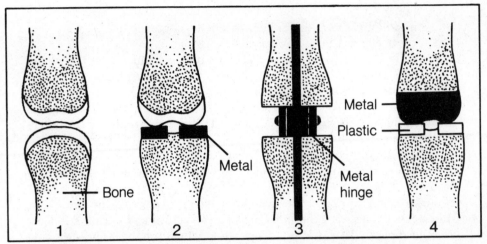

Knee arthroplasties: (1) normal knee; (2) partial replacement; (3) total replacement—hinge type; (4) total replacement

able designs in metal, plastic, and cement, for partial and total replacement (see diagrams). There is still some way to go before surgery on the knee produces the same level of results as on the hip but once more techniques are fast improving.

The same is true for slightly more experimental methods such as elbow, shoulder, ankle, and finger joint replacements, which have all been carried out with varying degrees of success. Among the noteworthy advances made in recent years is a revolving one-piece plastic finger joint developed by J. S. Calnan of the Hammersmith Hospital in London. This has enabled quite a few RA sufferers to have one or two crippled finger joints replaced in the space of only one day in the hospital. The patient comes in for the operation in the morning, has a new joint inserted under local anesthetic, and can be ready to go home at lunchtime. The actual surgery on the joint takes approximately twenty minutes–"Rather like going to the dentist," says Professor Calnan, "but less painful and worrying."

Another exciting development of recent years comes from Dr. Andrea Cracciolo of the University of California at Los Angeles, who claims good results with her replacement surgery for arthritic feet. She has used silicone implants—rubber toes—on forty-one patients, all of whom were unable to walk with any degree of comfort beforehand. After the operation, most of the arthritics could go back to walking and, what is very important psychologically, wearing smart shoes. More than thirty have had complete pain relief. One-fifth of all RA starts to affect the feet first of all, so this is clearly an important step forward in more ways than one. It has always struck me as ironical that the successes of hip and knee replacement surgery, though initially thrilling, are marred by feet that are too painful to walk on. So let us hope that other orthopedic surgeons will try to extend foot surgery along these or similar lines.

With the undoubted successes of joint replacement at the top of the orthopedic surgery list, it is all too easy to forget that there are in fact other operations which have been carried out to considerable effect. There is, for example, *synovectomy*, or the removal of the diseased and inflamed lining or synovium of the joint. This is appropriate for RA sufferers, but usually only when a single joint has deteriorated in a more pronounced fashion than the others. As with a number of measures available in medicine, the results from synovectomy are not unequivocal. The operation has been performed on a number of people who report that it eliminates pain. However, the synovium will regrow within the joint again after a few weeks, and the inflammation can return and with it stiffness. So unfortunately it cannot be an operation which produces sure-fire outcomes of a permanent nature.

A procedure for treating osteoarthrosis-type degenerative conditions goes by the name of *debridement*, which has been described as "spring cleaning" the joint to remove unwanted bony growths or loose pieces of bone and cartilage in the joint cavity. These may produce considerable pain and restriction of movement, so surgery consists literally of cleaning up the joint and smoothing out the irregularities.

Osteotomy is a procedure to realign a deformed joint, in which a piece of bone is removed and the joint reset. This is particularly relevant for those conditions where one part of a joint surface has worn away excessively or where a bad alignment or deformity has occurred. Even quite a small realignment can reduce pain substantially, but not all joints are suitable for the procedure.

Resection is the removal of bones. It sounds a slightly crude technique, and certainly it is among the older surgical procedures for arthritis. But it can be effective in the foot and the wrist.

Sometimes—not often—it is felt necessary to try to increase the stability of a joint, and curiously enough, this is done by stiffening it permanently. The operation is called *fusion* or *arthrodesis* and is designed to make a joint pain-free and strong at the expense of flexibility. Here we are back to one of those medical equations I mentioned earlier. It can be better to have a stiff wrist or knee and be free from pain than to keep mobile in agony. Occasionally fusion is done for hips and the back. It is a procedure with limited application but now and then has its uses.

Some joint pain, in the fingers or wrist, for example, may be produced by pressure on the nerves controlling particular limbs. There may have been injury, too, causing nerve fibers to grow in anomalous ways, producing pain more or less constantly. In cases such as these, neurological surgery can be tried, often to good effect. Nerve pressure can also produce back problems and result from one of a number of abnormalities in the disks or the spinal canal. Again, surgery is possible but fairly rarely carried out. It is not always successful. The advice of Dr. James F. Fries on the question of such operations is unequivocal: "You should avoid back surgery if you can, and it's mainly up to you."

Doctors, too, prefer to avoid back surgery if possible. Sciatica, for example, produced when a spinal disk slips out of line and presses on the sciatic nerve, may be treated by rest and manipulation. Until fairly recently, a major surgical operation was necessary if this treatment failed. However, it has been found that the fruit of the South American papaw tree contains an enzyme called chymopapain, which can be injected into the spine, where it digests away the protruding section of disk, thus relieving pressure on the nerve. Positioning the needle takes a good deal of care, but once it is in place properly, the papaw jab is reported to produce a 60 percent success rate—the same as surgery. Actually this particular treatment is not that new, having been tried first in 1963. What *is* new is the fact that in Britain, at least, it has been given official approval on grounds both of efficiency and safety. So it seems like a viable alternative to surgery, even if at first sight the use of papaw has a flavor of folk medicine about it!

Most people seek or are recommended surgery for arthritis because they are in pain or because the lack of joint mobility is interfering with their everyday lives. Some sufferers, a small minority it is true, are more concerned with the *cosmetic* benefits of surgery, looking to it as a way of improving their appearance. I can understand this. I have nothing whatsoever against trying to keep looking good by whatever means. But a word of warning. Orthopedic surgeons are not magicians. They can improve the appearance of an awkward-looking joint to some extent, but patients are sometimes disappointed by their efforts—probably because they were laboring under the delusion that looking good equals feeling good. It does not.

My personal experience of surgery for arthritis could have been more extensive than it is, had I taken my doctor's advice. But I did not. What happened was that a tendon in my left hand spontaneously ruptured. It was a tendon attached to the muscle that extends the thumb, so as a result my left thumb was permanently turned down. It did not really interfere with my work. There are very few movements in surgery and even fewer in research in which one needs to extend the thumb, I found, so I simply did nothing about the tendon. Sometime later I went to see a doctor friend of mine to have a general checkup and he looked at this and said, "When did this happen? Why didn't you have something done about it?" Next I went to an orthopedic surgeon, and he said he couldn't repair that tendon again, for it had retracted too far. But he would be able to take a tendon from the index finger and transplant it. Then I had a splint made, which I had to sleep with at night, and it pulled this finger up. It was made of aluminum, but it was very awkward to wear in bed. I used it one night, then threw it away. So when people ask me about surgery for arthritis I cannot help feeling how ironical it is that I, of all people, should have been slow to opt for a surgical option. Perhaps doctors really do make bad patients!

LIVING WITH PAIN 6

Pain is a universal experience. Rich or poor, old or young, male or female—every category, clan, type, sort, and branch of the human species has its share of pain. As we saw earlier, this is not simply mankind's misfortune, because pain is a warning signal that something is amiss and therefore a cue to take action. Put your hand by accident on a hot stove, and the sharp, burning sensation is a prompt, unequivocal notification to remove your hand as speedily as possible, which of course you do. Imagine how hazardous life would be *without* pain. Think of those mercifully rare individuals whose pain-sensitivity mechanisms are nonexistent. If they drink something too hot, they will not feel it scalding the inside of the mouth. If they lean accidentally on a rusty nail, it may enter their skin, carrying a dangerous blood infection before they are even aware of it. If some malfunctioning in the abdominal region or the head fails to produce a pain reaction, they may continue to walk around unknowingly when they should be examined by a doctor. Pain, in short, is an essential aspect of our natural bodily defense system—the early-warning radar, you might say, heralding an onslaught to come.

At the same time, pain is . . . well, painful, uncomfortable, agonizing, excruciating even, and all our instincts scream at us to be rid of it whenever or wherever it strikes. And, as one well-known actor once said during a TV show in Los Angeles, "Pain saps your strength." Without it you can better face the problems of living, you feel you are stronger physically as well as mentally. It may start mildly, as a vague twinge, an awareness that something is not quite right, and progress to a discomfort. Or it may pierce firmly and suddenly in an eye-blinking paroxysm, catching us unawares and gasping for relief. Small wonder, perhaps, that our primitive forebears often regarded pain as some supernatural visitation from evil spirits with imaginatively devilish ways of making us flinch.

As a doctor, I have long been familiar with pain of all degrees. It is, after all, an important diagnostic tool for locating and studying the nature of heart and other diseases. At medical school one is taught to respect pain. It is one of the doctor's key routes to understanding a patient's illness, and of course one of the major obstacles to a happy life for people who suffer from it. Pain, then, is both ally and enemy combined.

This paradoxical side of pain has always fascinated me, certainly long before I came to know pain intimately at first hand. Over the years I have made some observations that have helped me to understand it better.

First and perhaps most important is that the pain threshold—the point at which a stimulus turns from unpleasant to painful—varies enormously from person to person and within one person according to circumstances. A ten-year-old girl may not turn a hair when a syringe needle enters her arm, while her father, a powerfully built man, will wince appreciably. Then a week later that same man, with his apparently low pain threshold, will fight his way through blistering flames to rescue his child from a fire, and when he finally drags her out of the house he still seems unconcerned for his own pain, so anxious is he about his daughter's welfare.

Clearly, the extent to which we feel pain is not dictated solely by the severity of the painful stimulus. Subjective, circumstantial factors also come into play. This can lead to some bizarre observations. The American researcher Dr. Henry Beecher, as an officer in the U.S. Army during World War II, noticed that GIs suffering from incredibly ugly open wounds would seem oblivious of any pain. Yet, oddly enough, those wounded men would yell "like hell" when they saw a medical worker approaching with a syringe. Enormous pain from their wounds they could accept, but thoughts of the needle jab alarmed them! Another interesting observation came from Dr. Beecher's study of surgical patients who were expecting to receive the most powerful of all painkilling drugs, morphine. Instead, Dr. Beecher administered a totally inert substance, a placebo, which should have done nothing to relieve pain. In the event thirty-five out of one hundred patients found relief from the placebo. Their strong expectation that they were being given morphine was, it seemed, sufficient to bring relief.

Elsewhere there are many examples of the subjective and indeed problematical nature of pain: the dervishes who can pierce both cheeks with a sharp metal skewer, without appearing to feel any distress; wounded soldiers who can undergo quite major surgery without anesthetic, whereas they might, as we have seen, be sensitive to a needle; people who by virtue of religious or emotional affiliations seem to be able to lock into a pain-override mechanism, transcending the normal responses of their body. If we could understand a little of what is going on in these people, could we arthritis sufferers perhaps cope better with our pain? To some extent, I think we can, and presently I will be returning to the topic with a seven-point guide. Before doing so, however, I should like to look a little more closely at where pain really comes from and how it affects the arthritic in particular.

Theories about the nature of pain have been put forward for centuries, from supernatural explanations to Plato's view of "sharp atoms" pricking the body's atoms; but it was not until the Greek physician Galen started to dissect the bodies of animals to reveal the networks of nerves to their brains that the seeds of modern ideas began to be sown. Generations of doctors and scientists worked away at the problem of how we respond to pain. Some theories were firmly ousted by others as observational techniques for investigating the brain and its activities improved. There have also been a number of heated controversies, but in the twentieth century, and in particular the past twenty years or so, something approaching a consensus has begun to emerge, thanks to the influential "gate-control theory" of Patrick Wall and Ronald Melzack, who launched their ideas in the mid-1960s.

Briefly, the gate-control theory proposes that there is a "gate" in the spinal cord which decides how much pain feeling we have. Suppose you prick your finger. The signal travels from the receptor in your finger to the spinal cord's gate, where a set of nerve cells allocates an appropriate amount of pain, depending on the circumstances. The gate is a kind of neurological control post, receiving messages and apportioning weight to them before passing them up to the brain, where the pain sensation is registered. Different receptors handle potentially painful stimuli in different ways. A pin jabbed in the finger will cause an immediate pain. Prick the intestine, and there is no pain sensation.

So you can see that apprehending pain involves the complex neural and physical mechanisms of the gate-control theory, the properties of local pain receptors, and the subjective elements I discussed earlier. Mind and matter are inextricably interlinked in the process of responding to stimuli in a way we call "painful."

Among the circumstantial factors appearing to influence pain is the time of day, or rather night. Many arthritis sufferers experience the circadian effects I discussed in Chapter 2. Pain is frequently more acute in the small hours, when, as three British researchers wrote in *The Lancet* (Apr. 25, 1970), "the unoccupied mind has more time to dwell on the lack of progress in some chronic forms of therapy." The researchers, Hart, Taylor, and Huskisson, found that in RA, ankylosing spondylitis, and possibly degenerative joint diseases such as OA, and gout, the pain was worse early in the morning and at night than at any other time in the twenty-four hours. They cite the case of AS patients who are so stiff and painful in their spine on waking that it takes three to four hours before they are sufficiently mobile to be able to get dressed and ready for work. One person had to resort to setting his alarm clock at two- to three-hour intervals during the night, because otherwise the morning stiffness would simply be too much to overcome in order to go to work. I understand exactly how these people feel. I know when I get out of bed in the morning that I am going to have a lot of pain in my knees, back, and feet until I move around a bit; then the pain and stiffness disappear to some extent. This experience has been with me for so long now that I believe that when you have constant pain, you develop a higher threshold for pain. Because you know it's going to be there, you somehow condition yourself to accept it. Also, you appreciate the absence of pain much more than other people. It's like the story of the man who was sitting and bumping his head against the wall and somebody walking past says, "Why do you do that?" and he says, "Because I feel so much better when I stop." The same with pain; you feel so much better when the pain is less or when it is no longer there at all.

This is not to say that I have become in some mysterious way impervious to pain. Far from it. If I have managed to raise my threshold through constant practice, it still does not cushion me from pain generally. I much prefer to think of myself as trying to cope with and manage pain, rather than attempting to conquer or suppress it, at least on a permanent basis. Here, then, are my guidelines, which you may profitably exploit in your pain-relief campaign.

1. AIM FOR ACTIVITY WITHOUT FRENZY. During the course of a day I try to vary my activities as much as possible so that I never spend too long either sitting in a chair (or in the car) or subjecting my joints to vigorous activity. Were I to sit at my desk or around a committee table for several hours without stretching my legs, I know that my feet and knee joints would begin to stiffen. You may have found the same after watching TV or spending an enthralling evening at the theater or a concert. Afterward you feel a tightening and a growing awareness of a sensation turning to pain that only walking around or massaging the joint will dispel. Keeping a joint prone to inflammation too still for too long is usually asking for trouble, which is why many of us get that early-morning phenomenon I talked about earlier. Joints are designed to be moved, and even when there is relatively little inflammation, as with osteoarthrosis, they will become painful if kept still or in a fixed position, say at right angles when sitting in a chair or cramped up in a cinema seat.

Conversely, long operations used to impose considerable stresses on my feet and hands, just as trudging around a busy supermarket, carrying heavy loads, or even striding a lot on hard pavements (and that includes jogging) might do for you. In my case it was difficult, if not impossible, for me to take time out every hour or so, but that is what any arthritic should try to do if possible. Take a rest. Lift your feet to take the weight off them, preferably resting the knees straight, not bent. And be a little more thoughtful about how you bend and stretch to do even the most common-place jobs such as picking up something from the floor. It can be agonizing to squat down too quickly. Better still, try to arrange things around you so that you rarely have to bend or stretch for them. Suppose, for example, you often need to take objects from a drawer in a kitchen cabinet. Make sure that drawer is at waist height. Leave the more inaccessible drawers for those items of equipment you only take out once in a while.

2. EASE PAIN WITH HEAT. Although joint heat (calor) is one of the common symptoms in arthritis, warmth can be used to great effect therapeutically. On a cool day, a hot bath or shower can work a minor miracle to ease a painful back, knee, or shoulder. If you are planning to do a few exercises, warm up beforehand by soaking in a warm bath, or even just soaking the joints that are most painful, such as the fingers and toes. You can, alternatively, use a heat lamp or a hot-water bottle. Some doctors recommend a totally contrary method, namely ice packs or cold compresses to ease pain and produce an "afterglow" in which exercises can be done more easily. It is worth a try, but personally I, like most people, find that heat works better.

3. CONSIDER USING SOME KIND OF SUPPORT. Some cases of arthritis are helped by immobilizing a painful joint in a splint for a few days. The wrist in particular is one region where such a technique could be employed. Another is the back, where a brace, belt, or corset may give welcome support and relief. To be perfectly frank, I have not found this kind of aid especially useful. Metatarsal bars have helped support my feet during long operations, it is true, but so far at least I have not come across any other contraption that helped so much that I was prepared to put up with the inconvenience and, I fully admit, the feeling that it made me very visibly "disabled."

4. USE PAINKILLERS WITH PRUDENCE. At first sight, the role of painkilling drugs in arthritis would seem to be pretty clear-cut. Your hand or your knee hurts. You take a couple of aspirin or acetaminophen tablets. In fifteen to thirty minutes the pain begins to subside and, you hope, stop troubling you for several hours, perhaps longer. What is more, the drugs you have taken are cheap to buy and easy to acquire even in your local supermarket. So they must be safe, mustn't they? Why not, then, consider taking analgesics as a way of life, like putting milk in your coffee or sugar in your tea? We live in a pill-consuming society. Millions upon millions of them are consumed every day. At an aspirin symposium held in London at the Royal College of Surgeons in 1975, Dr. Gordon Fryers produced a staggering statistic: that an estimated 35,000 *tons* of aspirin were taken annually around the world, and of that total the comparatively

healthy little island of Britain accounted for no less than 1,500 tons—which is something like two tablets per person per week. Now, consumption on this near-astronomical scale can mean any of several things: that common drugs (of which I use aspirin as an example) are finding their way to everyone who needs them; or that some people are taking them in abnormally high quantities; or that everyone seems to have a pill-popping habit. My own view, having thought hard about the obvious increase in drug consumption in the past few years, is that the last explanation is probably the most accurate. We seem to have got into a behavioral pattern of reaching for "health-giving" chemicals to solve our problems, be they pain in arthritis or depression in divorce. We have tended to succumb to the lure of the admen and the pharmaceutical goodies they are peddling, so that we reach for the pill bottle unthinkingly whenever there is something not quite right. If we go to the doctor and he does not give us a prescription for medication in one form or another, we feel cheated, as if he has failed to recognize our ailment and our need. We have, in short, become addicts.

I am not saying that painkillers have no place in the treatment of arthritis, especially those which, like aspirin, have the added bonus of being anti-inflammatory in action. What I am saying, from my own experience as an RA sufferer, is that analgesics have a limited part to play. Even the most powerful painkillers (which can be addictive, an added deterrent) only mask the basic causes of arthritis and can produce considerable side effects if taken to excess. So use analgesics if you must, but do so as sparingly and as temporarily as you possibly can. Personally, I find them of no help to me. I prefer to get relief from anti-inflammatory agents, which brings me to point 5.

5. TRY ANTI-INFLAMMATORY DRUGS. Medicine is often called an art rather than a science, to emphasize that it is impossible to lay down hard-and-fast rules of treatment which will suit everyone. Whatever the pharmaceutical companies say in advertising their products, a given drug will simply not suit everybody. Some patients will react better or worse than others to a particular tablet or bottle of medicine, just as people will differ in their reactions to food or a piece of sculpture. I have found it useful to experiment, with my doctor's help, with many of the quite long list of anti-inflammatory agents on the market. Some I have found effective in reducing swelling in the hands and feet, and with it the accompanying pain, but they produce unpleasant side effects on the stomach. So I would try something else which did not upset my digestion, because generally speaking anti-inflammatory medicines need to be taken on a regular basis. From time to time a very bad attack has driven me to injections of cortisone or cortisonelike drugs, which will often produce superb results. However, I

resist the temptation which many people might have of repeating corti-sone injections too frequently, because of their well-established side ef-fects. I keep them for times *in extremis,* and suggest you do the same.

6. AVOID INTROVERSION IF POSSIBLE. Some people are born more in-ward-looking than others. That is the nature of their personality and there is little they or anyone else can do about it. We all know the difference between the introvert and the extrovert. One is outgoing and sociable, ready to discuss ideas, thoughts, and feelings at any time. The other is more cautious about displaying emotion, about externalizing what is going on in his head. Now, in recent years this introversion/extroversion leaning in our personalities has been shown to be implicated in all sorts of behav-ior, including to some extent our perception of pain. According to Dr. Frank Dudley Hart in his paperback book *Overcoming Arthritis,** the person who tends to externalize and move his preoccupation away from the confines of self to the wider horizons of the world around him is less prone to feel the pains of swollen joints. He writes: "There is no doubt that an arthritic sufferer who is keenly interested in things outside himself needs fewer pain-killing tablets than one absorbed in his discomfort and with no outside interests. The best analgesic is an occupied mind. Being busy and interested is an escape from pain."

Of course, we do not choose our personalities, so if we are introverted by nature we may be at a slight disadvantage here. But that is all the more reason it seems to me to fight pain by throwing yourself into life as fully as you can. Drive and ambition, the will to win, or to join in with what others are doing can have surprising therapeutic effects. It is almost as if the body's capacity for feeling pain were being drained off into another direction, as if the energy expended by pushing oneself to be alert and occupied were somehow smothering the effects of an inflamed joint. Ac-tually there is, when you come to think about it, a parallel here between the arthritis sufferer and the celebrated Indian yogis who are masters of the art of diverting pain. These remarkable people can walk over hot coals or lie, stripped, on a sharp bed of nails without recourse to drugs to deaden the pain. Their secret seems to lie in their capacity to focus their mind on other things, diverting their attention outward from themselves. People who have been subjected to the most brutal torture report that they were able to transcend the excruciatingly painful experience by their attitude of mind, by thinking of a loved one, for example, or some other precious memory that swamped their present horrendous circumstances. Religious martyrs, too, are said to have died with a beatific smile on their faces, even as the flames licked around them.

*Published by Martin Dunitz, 1981.

In all these cases a mental transfer from inward to outward seemed to have an analgesic effect, just as a rugby player will spend the last thirty minutes of a match unaware that he has a fractured arm, so intent is he on winning. On many occasions I have overcome pain because I had something to do. Often when I wake up in the morning, I would dearly like to stay in bed because my joints are so painful, perhaps getting up gingerly in mid-morning to take a leisurely bath and have heat treatment before starting the working day. But for years I did not succumb to those feelings. If a patient was to be wheeled into the operating theater that morning at 8:30, I wanted to be there, scrubbed up and ready for perhaps six, eight, or twelve hours of work. It is not that I felt "the patient's need is greater than mine" (true though that often is) so much as the fact that unless I pushed myself to do things I knew I would quickly end up doing nothing at all. At which point one might as well quit life altogether, which is not what suits me—and, I suspect, not what suits you either.

7. LEARN TO REDUCE YOUR ANXIETY. Elderly people, knowing that they are approaching the end of their days, are not usually afraid of dying as such. They are really anxious about such questions as "Will I be alone or in a hospital?" "Will I have enough money for my relatives to give me a decent burial?" And so on. Something similar happened to me when my arthritis was diagnosed. I was not so much distressed at having RA as worried about what it would mean to my life. I turned over in my mind all manner of anxieties: about my ability to play cricket on the beach with my kids; about being able to go out and about with my wife, Barbara; about how much surgery I would be able to do and how far I would be forced to channel my energies into research. Asking my doctor brought only partial satisfaction. He could tell me how he thought my RA would progress in the strictly medical sense, but he could not wipe out with his reassurances all my anxieties, fears, irrationalities, and terrors about my future.

With my uncertainties has come a certain amount of depression. Although by nature I tend to have a sunny disposition, not prone to big swings of mood, there was no preventing a wave of depressing thoughts sweeping over me from time to time. No one, unless he or she is superhuman, can ever be rid of this kind of reaction to life's ups and downs once in a while, and I was no exception.

I have found that there seems to be a close link between anxiety and my perception of pain. The one rises or falls with the other. If I wake up one morning comparatively free from pain, the whole world seems brighter and those nagging anxieties do not enter my head. In short, there is a vicious anxiety-pain cycle which one must try to break. Some people might resort to the careful use of antidepressant drugs, but powerful though those are, I do not myself find them useful. It is too easy again to latch on to pills and thereby put one's feelings on automatic pilot. Personally I reckon it is better to cope with anxiety without such aids, if I possibly can. Which means doing two things:

First, work out precisely what it is that is worrying you. Then try to take each fear in turn and assess how far it is justified. Never wander around with a mass of anxieties all jostling for attention in your head. Divide and conquer.

Second, talk about your worries with people close to you. It could be a wife or boyfriend, a colleague or a relative. Or you may be able to articulate your fears to a professional trained to help you put them in perspective.

The mere act of carrying out either or both of these two measures can in itself be a pain-relieving exercise.

TIPS FOR EASIER LIVING 7

Having warned you in the last chapter of the evils of introversion so far as pain is concerned, I am now going to suggest quite the opposite strategy for managing your everyday life. To have arthritis—and I am not the first person to make this comparison—is like being in a perpetual state of war, sometimes under direct attack, sometimes enjoying (if that is the word) a brief truce, most often engaged in various skirmishes with the enemy. Now, in war it pays to subscribe to the old Boy Scout's motto, "Be prepared." As an arthritic I have sat down calmly and analyzed my strengths, weaknesses, ambitions, and limitations. This has meant carrying out a kind of mental stocktaking of my total lifestyle: at work, at home, and at leisure. It has meant assessing the enemy and when it is likely to strike. At what time of day and in what kind of circumstance do I seem least protected?

Those of you who have read my book *One Life* (New York: Macmillan, 1970) will know that since my earliest days as a doctor, I have always been motivated by a desire to improve the quality of life. It has always seemed to me preferable to try an experimental procedure such as heart-transplant surgery than to watch another human being's existence rapidly ebb away in misery and despair. Of course, the operation can fail, or the post-op procedures of suppressing rejection can be unsuccessful. But at least one is doing something positive, not just waiting for the inevitable. Fatalism has no place in medicine.

This has been my professional philosophy, which I have carried over into my life as a patient. In fact, "patient" is not really a good term to describe me. I tend to be highly *im*patient with the restrictions that rheumatoid arthritis has increasingly imposed on me, and react to them with counteroffensive measures.

At home, for example, where one can to a great extent control the environment, I see no reason why everything should not be geared to my needs. An obvious but often overlooked example of this is the electrical supply to lights and power sockets. Why make it a fumbling nuisance to flick tiny switches or stoop to plug in a television when pull cords and waist-level outlets can easily be installed? Why not replace ungraspable slimy doorknobs with lever-type handles, or have a simple handrail fitted on stairs or in the bathroom where you know your hips or knees always give you trouble?

I am not suggesting that you get yourself into debt by having, say, an electric elevator installed. Nor that you should turn your house or apartment into a mad inventor's paradise. But think sensibly about your everyday habits and design your domestic milieu to suit you. Do not make a virtue out of laboring on in an alien, ill-fitting environment just because you do not want to admit to yourself that you have special needs. Everyone has special needs of one sort or another. Yours just happen to be those of the arthritic.

Think carefully, then, about some of these key activities.

SITTING

Look for a chair which is comfortable while giving full support to the back, perhaps with arm rests. Be careful, if your knees are stiff, not to have it too low, or you may have trouble unbending to get up. There are specially made chairs available which will help to raise you from a sitting to an upright position by means of a mechanical device. If you regularly sit at a table to write or type, fit it with good-quality casters so that you can swing it away from you easily when getting up.

BATHING AND GROOMING

The bathroom can be an extremely difficult area in the house. Apart from having special items of equipment installed, such as steps to help you in and out of the bath, you may be able to follow my example and develop your own coping techniques. One in particular came to me from an unexpected quarter.

Some years back my daughter Deirdre showed great promise in water skiing, did very well at it, and ended up representing her country overseas when she was twelve years old. Later on she came in third in the world in Australia and won the Australian water-skiing championship for women three times. I was training her, and I remember that often when we had to push the boat out in the water I was totally hampered by the pains in my hands. After a while, it got so bad that I knew that either I had to find a way to push the boat with less pain—or my boat-pushing days were numbered. So I began to move my arms and shoulders in slightly different ways, experimenting with movement, you might say.

I think the main thing was having tremendous ambition and drive—the pains that I had never really prevented me from doing what I wanted to— and the reason for this is that I learned to compensate for the pain by having different movements and using different muscles. For example, at the moment I have very bad arthritis in both wrist joints and I find it very difficult to bathe because I cannot push on my hands to lift myself up or let myself down. Therefore, I use my elbows to get in and out of the bath. This is how I compensate for this particular deficiency. There are other limitations imposed by severe arthritis in both wrist joints. Any movement requiring me to push myself up with my hands, using my wrists, I have had to avoid. Because my elbows and, at first, my shoulder joints were not affected, I have used them to get from a sitting or lying position into a standing position. Getting out of a chair, I also have to use my elbows.

You will find that anybody with some defect in movement uses what we call trick movements. A very good example of this was my wife, Barbara (now my ex-wife, I am sorry to say). The two of us had a very severe motor accident in which I broke a lot of ribs and she developed an injury of the brachial plexus. As a result, she had partial paralysis of the right shoulder and couldn't put her right hand behind her head when she fixed her hair. Well, what she does is use the left hand to bring the right hand into position, but it's done in such a very unobtrusive way that no one really notices it. There are quite a lot of examples of trick movements—learning to use a part that has not been damaged or not in pain to make the other part work. I have one such trick in the morning when I shave. When later on I developed a pain in my shoulder joints and especially in my right shoulder joint, it was very painful to bring the razor up to my chin. So I would use my left hand to bring the razor up.

WORKING IN THE KITCHEN

The kitchen can be a source of considerable trouble. Ovens never seem to be at the right height. There is a lot of stooping and stretching to do and so on. Again, a little thought can help. Why not, for example, have one continuous work surface alongside the oven so that heavy pots and casseroles can be slid instead of lifted? As a surgeon, accustomed to using those long-handled hospital taps, I would reckon that these could be a blessing for the person with the typical arthritic hand and fingers. So why not make inquiries about having such taps installed? Or a tap turner fitted to your existing fixture. As for height, appliances such as refrigerators can be fitted at eye level, thereby releasing valuable floor space in an otherwise crowded room. Knobs on ovens, stoves, and so on can also be modified to suit the arthritic hand and not at great expense. I have also seen some ingenious inventions such as a tea or coffee pourer—the pot rests on a hinged platform which can be tilted, obviating the need for lifting.

AIDS AND GADGETS

On the subject of aids and gadgets, you may get some ideas from the following paragraphs, adapted from Peter Evans's useful book *Getting On*.

The help available in the form of aids and gadgets is almost too extensive to catalogue, ranging as it does from major items such as automatic stair climbers—necessitating structural modification to the home—to simple adaptations of existing objects such as toothbrushes or keys using materials readily available at low cost (or even free). Clearly the use made of the full armamentarium will depend on:

> The amount of help needed (never use a gadget that gives too much help)
> The money available
> The extent of free or subsidized equipment available in your locality
> How good you or someone close to you is at making things
> Inventiveness

One rule, however, needs to be observed: *Consult your doctor about using particular aids*. He may feel it would be better to exercise a limb, say, rather than adjust to infirmity by leaning on the benefits offered by a gadget, however ingenious.

Cooking and Eating Aids

Of the many devices available to facilitate food preparation and eating, here is a selection.

BOUGHT ITEMS

> specially designed knives, forks, spoons, mugs
> plate guards to prevent spillage
> suction egg cup
> wall can-opener
> one-handed potato peeler, whisk, tray
> nonslip tray
> milk saver (prevents boiling over)
> saucepan guard
> single-cup infusion heater
> jar opener
> potato masher (D-shaped)

HOMEMADE ITEMS

> cutlery grips
> cutlery handle enlargers
> nonslip chopping board and tray

teapot tilter (for pouring)
tap turner
clip-on apron (uses wire in place of strings)
enlarged saucepan-lid handles (wood)
jar lids (with wood block attached for ease of turning)
potato and fruit holder (for peeling)
padded spoon handle (use absorbent cotton and surgical tape to enlarge
    grip)
handle enlargers (using rubber bicycle handles)

Bathroom and Dressing Aids

Many bathroom devices have to be bought, but some can be made quite easily yourself. Dressing aids are usually fairly simple to make.

BOUGHT ITEMS

toilet and bathtub rails
toilet seat raiser (makes it higher and easier to sit on)
tip-up toilet seat
rubber nonslip safety mats
clip-on suspenders
self-supporting stockings
front-opening brassieres
elastic laces (no need to undo them)
long-handled shoe horn
nonslip soles

HOMEMADE ITEMS

wrist bands on towels (made of tape/elastic)
toothbrush extenders (aluminum tubing)
sock loops (pull them up with hooked stick)
slip-on tie (elastic around neck)
expanding cufflinks (elastic between links)
firm-grip hairbrush holder (elastic across back to slip hand through)
sponge on handle (use wooden coat hanger)
suction nail brush (sticks to basin)
tap turner (made of wood)
washing aid (a long-handled dish-washing sponge covered with a face-
    cloth)

Mobility Aids

The most commonly used aid to getting about is of course the walking stick. But how about going upstairs? One idea is to attach a wrist strap to the stick so that it hangs down while the climber pulls himself up by the banister. Another is a homemade walking stick and half-step arrangement. This is for steps that are very deep. The half-step is a wooden box, and the walking stick is attached. The climber lifts up the box at each step.

BOUGHT ITEMS

wheelchair
tip-up chair
baby carriage clips (to carry shopping bag on walker)
picker-upper (long-handled, spring-loaded tongs)

HOMEMADE ITEMS

chair casters
sloping ramps over steps (easier for some to climb)
rails by steps

Recreation Aids

A book rest is an obvious requirement for the reader, as is a page turner consisting of a rubber finger stall slipped on the end of a suitably cut stick. Large-print books and magnifying glasses (on stands) are also available. But the list of leisure aids goes considerably beyond these. Here is a selection, all homemade:

pencil or pen holder: a plastic lightweight golf ball
typing aid: fit rubber-ended pencils into two short lengths of broom-stick—ideal for fingers that aren't flexible
telephone dialer: a small walking-stick-shaped piece of clear plastic acrylic tubing (bend by dipping in boiling water) gets into the number holes very easily
page turner: try small plastic clothespins or paper clips to separate the pages
playing-card holders: a nylon scrubbing brush does it very well, or you can cut slots in a block of wood
needle stand: for threading, stick the needle into a broad cork stopper
darning stand: a wooden darning mushroom can easily be fitted onto a G-shaped clamp to hold it firm on a table
pipe-holder: for the person who cannot raise his arms, the pipe can be held at mouth level in a spring clip fixed to the end of a broomstick on a suitable base.

SLEEPING

The bedroom is ostensibly a place of rest and tranquillity, but in reality for many arthritis sufferers an area of discomfort and dismay. Good sleep is essential to us all, with or without joint problems, and whether we need a modest five hours per night or a regular eight or nine. Bed manufacturers often make great capital out of the fact that we spend so much of our lives in bed, and with justification. But whereas the nonarthritic can afford to some extent to turn a deaf ear to their attentions, I have found it important to choose my bed carefully. I need good support for the body from the mattress, and I like a low-slung bed so that I can swing out easily in the morning. In South Africa one has little problem keeping warm, but on cooler nights I have no hesitation in reaching for the bed socks or switching on the electric blanket. Sheets and blankets are, I find, a bit of a nuisance. So for years now I have used a good-quality comforter, which gives me total mobility in an unbroken cocoon of warmth.

MAKING LOVE

One aspect of life which I know worried me initially and bothers many other arthritis sufferers is sex. As far as I know, arthritis doesn't make a man impotent, but of course lovemaking itself, which can be very physical, is retarded by it. It gives you pain. Even during intercourse itself you will feel the discomfort. Although it's enjoyable, it is painful. If you find it difficult to have sex, try to discover other ways of making love in which there's not so much activity. To be frank, I have found that arthritis and the pain it causes have at times interfered with how well I can make love. If an arthritic man lies on top of a woman and rests on his elbows, this can produce pain in the elbow joint. So maybe he has to lie sideways. Sometimes you have got so much pain that it is such an effort to get going on the sexual scene that you think, "Oh, I will just leave it." It helps if your partner is understanding of your deficiencies. The nonsufferer has to understand the other's problems and help him or her to compensate for them. Try to compensate in a way that does not put undue demands on you or the other person. Choose positions that you know are not going to be difficult, and try to vary your style of making love so that it will be easier for your partner. For example, if a man has the sort of arthritis that I have, I would advise his wife, "You must now try to be the leader, the one who initiates love and try and work up passion instead of passively waiting for your man to be the dominant character. You should become the more active one."

Arthritis should never be the reason for two people not to make love. I remember once seeing a documentary on television about a man who had become paralyzed from his neck down—not, apparently, the sort of individual likely to enjoy sex anymore. But when questioned on this intimate aspect of his marriage, he grinned mischievously and said, "Oh, well, one can do quite a lot still, you know. Ask my wife!"

DRESSING

You can make life less stressful for yourself by wearing clothes that are loose-fitting, comfortable, and easy to slip on and off, fasten and unfasten.

Zippers beat buttons, and Velcro-type fasteners can be so much more convenient than, say, snaps. Avoid any clothing, including footwear, that directly aggravates your arthritis. It is not necessary to endure pain in a
masochistic route to high fashion. For a woman with arthritic feet to
squeeze them into high heels is understandable but wrongheaded. If you
can put a good-looking outfit together that involved stiletto heels, you can
surely do the same with something less detrimental to the health of your
joints!

DRIVING

One everyday activity which every arthritis sufferer soon learns to consider carefully is driving. Here you have to make sure that you can get in
and out of the door reasonably easily—from the passenger as well as driver's side if there is heavy traffic on the street. You also need well-
positioned controls such as gear shift and steering wheel, and a driving
seat position which enables you to keep your knee joint at a fairly shallow
angle. Good hip and back support is vital, especially for longer journeys.
If you can get automatic transmission and power steering, you will find
that these will ease the driving burden.

A WORD ABOUT CHILDREN WITH ARTHRITIS

So far in this chapter the everyday problems of arthritis I have been
dealing with are those of adults. However, as we saw earlier, children get
arthritis, too. In Britain alone there are thought to be around 6,000 children, some as young as just one year old, who succumb to arthritis. Seven
out of ten, mercifully, make a complete recovery, but during their period
of illness and for the other 30 percent who do not recover, I sympathize
fully with parents and friends who want so much to find ways to alleviate
their suffering. Apart from surgery, which can produce superb results in
some cases, physiotherapy, exercise (under the doctor's watchful eye, of
course), and sometimes splints to prevent deformities are all useful.
Swimming will help maintain muscle tone and joint mobility, whereas
hard contact sports such as football or basketball can be damaging to joints
as a result of constant jarring, turning, and jumping. Probably the one
thing above all others that distresses parents of the arthritic child is that
feeling that their youngster is "different" from his or her peers. This can
show itself in all sorts of ways, not only exclusion from sporting activities
but being left behind in the classroom when the disease is active and
prevents attendance at school. So discuss with your child's teachers ways
of keeping him or her up to date. Think of ways of keeping the young
patient in the social swim as much as possible, to break down that "out-

sider" syndrome. Children are extraordinarily adaptable and naturally compassionate with their weaker brethren, provided they are totally familiar with their problems. Never try to hide arthritic children away to protect them from the ravages of life. This ends up producing precisely the opposite effect to that which you originally intended.

ALTERNATIVE THERAPIES   8

When people started to learn of my rheumatoid arthritis, they began to write suggesting their favorite remedies. After a time the trickle turned into a flood, and my secretary was swimming around in hundreds of unusual arthritis treatments. Everybody, it seemed, wanted to cure me. Well, I collected these "cures" from all around the world and compiled a catalogue of lotions, potions, and notions which I call my "arthritis album."

The metal cures alone would have turned me into the original bionic man with metal and zinc heels on my shoes, copper bracelets on each arm, copper pennies taped to the right leg (above the ankle, to be exact) and a nickel coin on the left. Then there was the alpha cure, derived from an electric current which amplifies the alpha waves of the brain and feeds them into pulse generators. The generators are applied above and below the afflicted joint and are claimed to have completely cured a ninety-seven-year-old rheumatism sufferer. It was just possible that I could have got away with a grand entrance to the operating theater, metal heels tapping, coins clinking, and bangles jangling, while pulse generators hummed quietly at each wrist, if somebody hadn't already created a sendup of the whole costume. They even gave it a name—and put it in a film called *Star Wars*.

Natural cures were legion. I liked the suggestion from a British sufferer who recommended gin, but I found the required mixture of sulfur and lemons a bit much, as were oil of rosemary and raspberry tea. Green tomato juice and dried papaw seeds seemed acceptable, but what about vitamin E oil and halibut capsules?

Someone from South Africa added chemicals such as Kruschen salt, calcium, and a number of more exotic compounds, topping it all with an electric blanket. Other ideas from my fellow countrymen were parsley, celery, blackstrap molasses, khaki bush leaves, controlled breathing, sun baths, sisal juice, chiropody, honey and queen bee jelly, cane liquor (ah, that's better), saltpeter, bitter blaar leaves, and transcendental meditation.

I particularly liked one individual who swore by a well-known make of dog pills—but I couldn't help wondering about all those aging pooches to be seen lolloping arthritically on any beach!

Also recommended were two types of brand-name brake fluid with elaborate instructions about the container and the length of overnight joint soaking to be done. In the same category were injections of olive oil into the joints, along with morning pushups and "boxer's jabs." The marriage of mechanical know-how and medical practice was also attempted in the suggested use of a patent rust remover and solvent for freeing nuts and bolts.

An arthritic in Kenya came up with lotions of boiled guava leaves, and a Zimbabwean advised rubbing the joints with brass polish—a course of treatment which, even if it had not succeeded, might have given me the cleanest knuckles in the West.

Indonesians opted for ultraviolet rays. A man in Singapore sent a bracelet made from a submarine plant growing on rock coral, and Malaysia offered papaw and meat soup. (A nice echo of that sciatica injection I mentioned earlier.) Indians produced a long list which included yoga, herbal medicines, and homeopathy.

Ireland solemnly affirmed the use of stinging nettles and acupuncture. Holland agreed on the herbal remedies. Italy suggested several oils. Germany offered an armory of respected pharmaceuticals, and so did the Dominican Republic. Canada came up with its famous balsam, alfalfa, more pharmaceuticals, a diet of beeswax and gelatine, herbal tea and lemon.

Costa Rica added to the herbal cure list. Brazil was for naturally occurring radioactive springs, while Argentina named mineral springs, an oral vaccine, amino acids, vitamins, and drugs. A woman in Puerto Rico wanted me to try lemon and honey, and burial in hot sand, though not at the same time.

From Australians came a recommendation for eucalyptus oil, though they hedged what looked like a good bet with salts, herbs, and drugs. Someone from New Zealand guaranteed that country's sulfur springs.

The United States knew exactly what their rheumatics needed, and righteously said so, beginning with heated vibrators, plaster of Spanish fly, whirlpool baths, fresh cherries, and—inevitably—peanut oil. They also suggested Scientology, green plastic hair curlers on the affected fingers to act as "pain filters," burdock root, and osteopuncture.

Shakespeare would have liked the American who suggested blood from a baby's umbilical cord, centrifuged to obtain the plasma and administered by injection.

I liked the twelve-year-old Oregon boy whose reaction to his mother's description of my illness was a spontaneous: "Gosh, that makes me feel sad," and the writer who said that a potato in every pocket would do the trick.

What impressed me most of all was the feeling that there was lots of love in every one of those letters, no matter how curious, cranky, or comic the suggestions put forward. They were sent without thought of reward and with one purpose, to help someone they had never seen and were unlikely to meet, a faraway stranger known only through the columns of a newspaper. I have always found it humbling to be the receiver of gifts, but to be the focus of so much care and spontaneous sympathy is an experience difficult to convey. The overall impression is one of enormous strength, a kind of warmth of the soul, and the feeling that, given the chance, people everywhere actually like each other and want to be liked in turn.

To be perfectly honest, I found the affection contained in all those letters more valuable than the cures themselves. Some, in fact, I felt would be downright dangerous even to try. But it was as a result of reading people's suggestions—some clearly cranky, others perfectly respectable— that I began to develop an interest in what used to be called "fringe" practices. So now I should like to discuss the possible role in arthritis treatment of what people now prefer to describe as alternative medicine.

When I was a medical student (and I doubt that things have changed much in the intervening decades), to be a doctor was, we were taught, to put into practice the accumulated wisdom of orthodox scientists: the anatomists and physiologists who described the complexities of the body machine; the neurologists who tried to unravel the "enchanted loom" of the brain; the biochemists who showed how each of us is a finely tuned, individual chemical factory, manufacturing products to sustain us; and all the other "ologists" who have contributed to our understanding of how the body functions. As scientists they were, and are, clever but cautious men. Each effect, be it an illness or a remission, must have a cause. Treating diseases, they remind us constantly, is a matter of applying cool, calculating reason to our physical abnormalities or deficiencies and setting them to rights by observation-based logic.

Many centuries ago, on the other hand, it was believed, quite erroneously, that a sick person was someone whose bodily "humors" or vital essences were out of proportion. There were said to be four humors, and an imbalance among them of any kind would result in the symptoms of disease. This was before the days of experimental medicine, of dissecting dead bodies to find out what was wrong in their organs. A more mechanistic view of cause and effect had not yet begun to replace the vague, semireligious beliefs that prevailed. Now, the change of direction from the purely intuitive to the rational was of supreme importance in setting medicine on a "proper" scientific footing. Without it the astounding progress that has led to antibiotics, transplant surgery, the EMI scanner, and all manner of "miracles" would be inconceivable.

And yet something in me—and, it appears, in a growing number of people, both doctors and lay persons—says that modern scientific medicine, for all it has to offer, does not and probably *cannot* say it all. In fact, I have begun to wonder whether, by discarding all that does not clearly fit in with the facts as narrated in medical textbooks, we have not thrown out the baby with the bathwater.

When I first began to look seriously into the claims of the so-called alternative therapists, I was heavily skeptical. My training had seen to that. For me they represented a kind of updated medical mumbo-jumbo, a mixture of superstition, folklore, misplaced faith, and downright ignorance. Like many people, I had heard or read accounts of hoaxers and charlatans, pretending to be faith healers or psychic surgeons or concocters of healing potions. To put oneself in the hands of anyone but a skilled and, above all, orthodox physician seemed to be asking for trouble. From my own experience I knew that people will rapidly override their natural hardheadedness when it comes to seeking a "cure." They are often looking for a miracle, and they express their anxiety to find one by becoming completely irrational. They will try anything, however useless or absurd, in the faint hope that it will work for them or their loved ones. Now, I understand these feelings and have seen them in action many times. But my whole professional life tells me that most of these treatments are totally ineffectual as medical treatment. So, much as I sympathize with people who behave in this way, I could not honestly say that it is therapeutically productive, except in a psychological way, since it gives one a sense that one is doing *something*. Here, then, was the basis of my skepticism: a mixture of my medical training and my clinical experience.

Then came my arthritis—an incurable disease treatable to some extent, but still painful day in, day out. There were painkilling and antiinflammatory drugs to help me, as well as the other procedures I have discussed in earlier chapters, but some of these have their drawbacks: cortisone, for example, brings relief at the expense of undesirable side effects. At the time, the late 1960s, I was beginning to notice how often alternative treatments such as acupuncture, biofeedback, and homeopathy were creeping into medical discussions. More and more doctors seemed to be opening their minds to the possibility that what had so often hitherto been dismissed as suspect quackery could contain more than an element of genuine usefulness. Intrigued by this thought I began to read, discuss, and try to make up my own mind on the matter. I also, as you will read in a moment, tried one or two alternative therapies for myself.

My first problem was that of wheat and chaff. What really is an "alternative therapy" as opposed to a piece of superstitious nonsense? Take those cures sent in to me by well-wishers. Among them were suggestions that nowadays some rheumatologists and general practioners might recommend, though most were outrageously quackish. How could anyone assess critically whether a potential treatment is even worth trying? Even rheumatologists can have trouble at times sorting wheat from chaff, as illustrated by the following story told by leading expert Frank Dudley Hart in the *British Medical Journal* (27 March 1976). In 1951, when the newly discovered cortisone was being hailed as the arthritis wonder drug, some people were for one reason or another unable to obtain it. Then a researcher in Sweden declared that similar results could be obtained from another compound called deoxycortone (Doca) and ascorbic acid. What followed was an exercise in faith healing.

Such was the expectant electric atmosphere of the time that our outpatient clinic acquired a Lourdes-like quality. Patients who had not fully extended shoulders or elbows for many months dramatically did so, walked corridors briskly, and, in one case, jumped over the bed. The second injections had less impact, however, and the third failed to do any good whatsoever. A year later I asked one of these patients what treatment had ever done her any good? "None whatsoever!" "What about the double injections we gave you a year ago?" "They were no good at all!" "But this is what you wrote at the time and this is your own handwriting of a year ago: 'I haven't felt like this for years. It's a miracle. I have no pain and can move easily and freely.' What about that?" And looking rather hurt and baffled all she could say was "I must have been crazy at the time I wrote that." Crazy or not it worked while the enthusiastic heat was on, but what we got to know as the triple response to faith healing was the rule: excellent, fair, nil to first, second, and third treatments respectively. Only a few patients can maintain that continuous complete faith in the future that transcends pain and depression.

It seems there are a few patients, with arthritis and other diseases, who seem to benefit from *any* form of treatment, even if only temporarily. They will claim relief from pain by wearing copper bangles, say, or some other method which cannot possibly "work" in the accepted sense—though even as I write this, some people are claiming that the old copper bracelet talisman may in fact be releasing minute quantities of valuable trace elements through the skin. Such people may be using faith or some other inner resource to do the treatment for them. Remember that when a new drug is being tested, it is important that people taking it do so "blind"; that is, some patients are given the drug being tested while others receive an inert placebo. Otherwise their response to the drug may be influenced by the placebo effect one observes in giving anything resembling a pill or a jab. Dr. Dudley Hart, in his paperback book *Overcoming*

*Arthritis,** sums up the role of what we might call nonmedical factors in arthritis cures thus: "It is fair to say that almost any drug that has done any good in any other disorder has been tried in the treatment of rheumatoid arthritis, and if faith and optimism are present in either patient or doctor some good results will be obtained for a time in every case, the highest proportion occurring when abundant faith is present in both doctor and patient, particularly if the latter has complete faith in the former."

I can endorse the importance of faith and optimism from my own experience as a cardiologist and cardiac surgeon. I never like to operate on patients who say they are going to die, because they virtually always do die. Once I operated on a South African who had an aortic valve disease, and he said, "I am not going to make it. I am going to die." I did the operation, which was a straightforward aortic valve replacement, after which he went to the intensive care unit. Afterward, for the next two or three days, there was never any problem whatsoever. But he kept on saying, "I am going to die." Well, six or seven days later, on a Sunday afternoon, his family came to see him and he sat up chatting to them. Half an hour later, after they had left, the nurse came in to find him dead in his bed.

In another operation a child was wheeled into the operating room, and she kept crying, "I don't want to be operated on. I am going to die." I operated on her, and she died. So I am very superstitious on that score. I do believe that a person's attitude toward his disease and his real willingness to get better play a definite role in his recovery, and that is true whether the treatments being given are orthodox or unconventional.

To return to the question of alternative therapies for arthritis, below are those which I and other sufferers have investigated—in my case mostly on paper, in theirs by actually trying out the treatments available. For some of those methods I must say that I retain my skepticism, but being a sufferer has taught me that unless something is positively dangerous, there's no harm in trying anything. It may work for you, for reasons that I and possibly no one else can fully articulate.

ACUPUNCTURE

Acupuncture comes at the top of the list because it has received so much attention both inside and outside the medical profession in recent years. It is undeniably a fascinating technique to watch in action, with a history stretching back possibly five thousand years. The word means literally pricking (puncture) with a needle (from the Latin *acus*). No doubt through films and TV you are at least partly familiar with the use of fine needles inserted at various parts of the body and tweaked by the thera-

*Published by Martin Dunitz, 1981.

pists from time to time. The ideas behind this ancient Chinese form of practice are not easy for the Westerner to grasp because they seem to us to be a slightly bizarre marriage of medicine and quasi-religious belief, whereby the therapist tries to restore the balance of the individual's vital energy or *chi*, essential (so it is believed) to good health. The acupuncturist's technical diagrams show a criss-crossing network of lines or meridians, the invisible channels by which the *chi* is carried, with various points along the way at which needles can be inserted. Not necessarily at the part of the body affected by disease, I should add. With acupuncture, relief from illness in one region of the body may be produced by insertion of a needle elsewhere.

Actually, arthritis has for some time been a target for needle-pricking treatments. It used to be quite common in the last century to plunge a needle into the affected joint to try to find relief, but it is really only in the last twenty to thirty years that the traditional Chinese techniques have begun to gain anything like a foothold. The attitude of the medically orthodox, though, is still often quite unbending. "Lunacy" is how one eminent pharmacologist has described acupuncture. Others are less emphatic. One eminent rheumatologist, for example, says that there is evidence that acupuncture can relieve pain, perhaps by somehow activating the body's system for manufacturing its own morphine-like substances, the endorphins (the discovery of which was undoubtedly one of the most exciting pieces of brain research in this century).

What use, then, is acupuncture in rheumatic and arthritic disorders? Well, fortunately, the British Arthritis and Rheumatism Council has helped to answer that question by asking two doctors—one a skeptic and the other an advocate of the technique—to air their views on paper. The results were published in two articles in the council's journal, and I reproduce most of them below for you to make up your own mind.

First the view of the sceptic, Frank Dudley Hart in an ARC publication:

> . . . What conditions are said to benefit most [from acupuncture]? According to Yoshio Manaka and Ian A. Urquhart in *The Layman's Guide to Acupuncture*, published by Weatherhill, New York, in 1972 (p. 126), group A (the best) are headaches, muscle pains, cramps and depression. Group B (second best) includes diarrhoea, painful periods, shingles and "rheumatism" (but they do not define this last disorder). Group C—inconstant (uncertain) arthritis, asthma, diabetes mellitus, angina pectoris. Group D (symptomatic improvement only)—tuberculosis, cancer, Parkinson's Disease, hemiplegia, infantile paralysis.
>
> From this list it would appear that mild disorders, which get better naturally with encouragement, do best and this is borne out by what many patients have told me. Very few bad rheumatoid sufferers, in my experience, derive any lasting worthwhile benefit. But milder, transient

conditions in patients who do not like or get no benefit from drugs or cannot tolerate them, sometimes do.

Nobody with tuberculous disease or diabetes would think of relying on acupuncture alone as there are very adequate treatments available. Many patients have symptoms which worry them and cause discomfort and some distress, but which are not based on serious underlying disease. Such patients do sometimes benefit considerably from acupuncture as they often do from a number of medicines, physiotherapy or other forms of treatment.

Time cures

Time cures most disorders, for most disorders, even disc backache and frozen and painful shoulders, get better naturally given time, and whatever is given during this time gets the credit. The longer that treatment is continued the more likely is the cure to be seen. Very often it is not the acupuncture, the physiotherapy, the manipulations, the drugs or anything else, but Mother Nature herself, hand in hand with Father Time, who is responsible but seldom gets the credit.

Nevertheless acupuncture does undoubtedly relieve painful symptoms and helps in easing the aches and pains of a number of arthritic conditions, though not permanently curing the underlying disorder or altering the natural course of the disease. It would seem on present evidence to be, like physiotherapy, a symptom relieving physical method given while nature effects the cure. Shiatsu, literally finger pressure, is a Japanese form of finger massage and pressure, usually applied by another member of the family, which does with the fingers what basically is done by the acupuncturist with his needles. The so-called do-in is Shiatsu done by oneself with one's own finger.

What is seldom mentioned in articles on acupuncture is the possible complications of this form of therapy; it is a truism of medicine that any form of treatment that can do good can on occasion do harm.

In *An Outline of Chinese Acupuncture*, . . . reference is made to them. Dizziness, faint feelings and actual fainting turns may occur as they may with any needling. But also puncture of the lung, the kidney, the spleen, the liver, the pericardium and, rarely, brain and spinal cord with convulsions, paralysis and coma, when immediate emergency measures have to be taken. These are undoubtedly extremely rare but are reported, and the possibility of transmitting viral hepatitis is a real one unless autoclaving [sterilizing] is done. For simple cleansing of needles with alcohol or any other antiseptic will not prevent this.

In general, however, complications with acupuncture as performed for the usual forms of arthritis are extremely rare.

Now to the unequivocal advocate of acupuncture in arthritis, Dr. Felix Mann, who interestingly enough studied under Dr. Dudley Hart at London's celebrated Westminster Hospital. Dr. Mann is something of a pioneer in the use of acupuncture for arthritis, having practiced it since the late 1950s. Like many pioneers, he has received his share of abuse and derision from colleagues. Here are his views:

Acupuncture has a certain, though perhaps limited, effect in the treatment of the general group of rheumatic disorders. In some conditions the results are good, in others useless. It is therefore important to know how to pick the likely winners.

Fully developed osteoarthritis and rheumatoid arthritis involve physiological and anatomical changes in the body which are more or less irreversible. The damage to the bone in both conditions is often so great that the body cannot regrow to the previous healthy state.

If one's skin is cut with a knife, it will normally regrow to practically its former state. If one has a hole in a tooth, no amount of dentistry or medicine will heal that hole; instead, a dentist fills it with amalgam or other substance.

Eroded

In developed rheumatoid and osteoarthritis the bone inside the joint and the cartilage have been eroded. This eroded tissue, as holes in teeth, is a type of tissue which has no regenerative ability and hence cannot regrow, or if at all, only to a small extent.

For the above reason acupuncture cannot effect a fundamental cure; nor for that matter are drugs very helpful. Drugs may partially overcome this impasse by relieving pain, reducing the inflammatory response of the joint, relaxing appropriate muscles etc.

Acupuncture may on rare occasions help an irreparably damaged joint. One has the impression that this occurs by relaxing the muscles around the joint, so that the roughened areas of bone are not crammed together by muscles in spasm. Thus the relaxed muscles prevent the bones from grinding on one another.

However, electrical tests on the activity of muscles around joints have been performed, disproving this theory: when the pain in the patient was reduced by acupuncture, the muscle activity was neither increased nor reduced.

Acupuncture is normally of no help in a patient with active rheumatoid arthritis: when the joints are warm, the blood sedimentation rate is raised more than a small amount, the patient is anaemic and feels generally ill as if recovering from 'flu. The possibility of help usually only arises in a "burnt out" rheumatic, when the active process has largely or even completely declined, and also if the resultant damage to the joints, as mentioned above, is only fairly minimal.

Neck Pain

Pain in the neck (Cervical Spondylosis) may, in the milder case, be frequently helped by acupuncture.

If the degenerative changes in the vertebrae of the neck are severe, acupuncture will either not help, or help only a minimal amount, or only help temporarily.

If the degenerative changes in the vertebrae are mild, the chances of acupuncture being helpful are greater.

The "easier to treat" cases will have only mild restriction of neck movement; pain limited to the neck, shoulder or back of the head; and symptoms which are not constantly present.

The failure rate is considerably higher if there is a greater restriction of neck movement; if the pain goes down the arm or to the hand and fingers; if there is wasting of the muscles of the hand; if the fingers feel dead or there are anaesthetic areas of skin; or if the strength of the hand is more than fractionally reduced. An X-ray of the vertebrae of the neck is of less use in deciding the probable outcome of treatment, than a careful appraisal of the patient's symptoms.

Lumbago

Lumbago and Sciatica may (as shown in most of the above examples) be helped in the milder case.

If there is a genuine "slipped disc" (supposedly only 5% are genuine) acupuncture does not help. If the patient has severe osteoarthritis of the vertebrae in the lower back, again acupuncture is of no avail. There are also several, somewhat rarer, diseases of the vertebrae or spinal cord, where acupuncture is powerless.

A sudden severe attack of lumbago or sciatica, in which the patient cannot move and is locked in position, is usually unsuitable for acupuncture. It is better treated by bed rest, sometimes drugs or manipulation, and on rare occasions with an operation.

The mild, long continued, lumbago or sciatica is not infrequently better treated by acupuncture. Once someone has back trouble, the weakness will remain for life, unless they are lucky. However acupuncture may, not infrequently, ameliorate the trouble to a worthwhile extent, though unfortunately these patients may need a single "pep up" treatment on rare subsequent occasions. A knowledge of which movements are harmless and which are to be avoided and an appropriate bed, are just as important as acupuncture in the long term management of such patients.

The chances of success are considerably diminished (as in neck pain) if the pain is constant twenty-four hours of the day, day after day, week after week; if there is more than slight wastage of muscles (unless this is merely due to not using them); if there are dead areas or the skin is anaesthetic; if the muscles become excessively weak; or if there are gross circulatory changes.

Other conditions

Other conditions where acupuncture may help vary considerably— pain in the knee, big toe joint, shoulder, wrist, etc., may all respond, but usually only if the damage to the joint is fairly minimal. Osteoarthritis of the hip joint, except in rare instances, responds only temporarily.

Speed of Response. Probably half the patients who eventually benefit from acupuncture notice some improvement of their symptoms within a few seconds or minutes of the first treatment taking place. The remainder respond a few hours or days later, or on very rare occasions, two weeks later. Some patients need two or three treatments to notice the initial response. A fully qualified doctor, who knows orthodox medicine and acupuncture, will often have a reasonable idea of the chance of success from the first treatment.

Mechanism

Acupuncture exerts its influence, at least to some extent, via the physical nervous system. This is illustrated by the fact that if the nerve which leads from the pricked area of skin to the spinal cord is somehow severed, the acupuncture has no effect. Likewise if the function of the nerve leading from the spinal cord to the diseased part of the body is disrupted the acupuncture fails. The same applies with parts of the spinal cord or the involved parts of the sympathetic nervous system.

The role played by the naturally occurring pain inhibitors, the endorphins and enkaphalins, is less certain. The lower and higher centres of the brain, psycho-somatics and many other factors, are probably also involved.

And there I will leave acupuncture, except to point out that if you do feel you would like to try it, make absolutely sure that you are treated by a properly trained and qualified practitioner. Look for guidance both from your regular doctor (if he is prepared to give it) or organizations such as the Arthritis Foundation.

If you try acupuncture, I hope you have more success than I did. Once, out of desperation, I went to a medically qualified doctor in Cape Town who practiced this form of alternative medicine. I undressed to my underpants, noting that there was no attempt to sterilize the many needles which were inserted into my feet, ears, and arms, until, looking like a porcupine, I stood there while the therapist said, not terribly encouragingly I thought, "This either works or it doesn't." It did not. Worse than that, the next day I felt the most excruciating pain I had ever experienced. So much for acupuncture for yours truly.

HOMEOPATHY

Another unorthodox therapy which has been proposed for arthritis for many years is homeopathy. Its remedies derive from herbs and minerals which have been used to treat illnesses for centuries, though the manner of dispensing them is at first sight a little paradoxical. Instead of treating a disease with drugs that counter the symptoms, as in administering aspirin to lower fever or reduce inflammation, the homeopath gives substances which normally would actually produce the symptoms complained of. What is more, whereas conventional drug therapy involves giving higher doses the more serious the ailment, homeopathic remedies are more powerful when extremely diluted. The idea is to "treat like with like," but by adopting a very special procedure for preparing the homeopathic remedy. The substance is first diluted, sometimes to one part in a billion; then the mixture is shaken rapidly—"succussed" is the technical term. The ensuing compound can be taken in liquid form or as pills, powders, granules, or ointments. The potency of the remedy and the frequency with which it is taken are a matter for the practitioner to decide, in consultation with the patient—not unlike conventional drug therapies.

The medical establishment has often denounced homeopathy as "unscientific." How, it is asked, can these minimal amounts of active substances have any appreciable therapeutic effects? Well, the only way to test homeopathy's claim is to submit it to experimental investigation, which in the medical world means carrying out a "blind" trial, whereby one drug is tested against another in a controlled setting, with no one—neither patients nor doctors—knowing which person is receiving which drug until the results are in.

One such trial was carried out in a collaborative effort in Glasgow, where doctors from the Homeopathic Hospital, the Centre for Rheumatic Disease, the university's Department of Medicine, and the Royal Infirmary got together to study the use of homeopathy in rheumatoid arthritis. The patients, ninety-five in all, had suffered from RA from a matter of months to many years. They were divided into two groups. Fifty-four were given a homeopathic remedy, while forty-one were treated with aspirin, the old standby for inflammatory disease. At the end of the trial, twenty-four of the homeopathically treated were better; six were better with aspirin. The dropout rate for homeopathy was 33 percent, compared with 85 percent for aspirin, many through adverse side effects. So this one trial seemed to say something positive about homeopathy and RA.

On the other hand, quite recently the *Lancet* published a similar study in which a homeopathic remedy for osteoarthrosis was compared with a standard anti-inflammatory agent and analgesic, fenoprofen, and an inert substance (placebo) with no chemical action. Again the trial was a collaborative effort, involving the Royal London Homeopathic Hospital, two other hospitals, and the Department of Rheumatology at King's College, London. The homeopathic remedy used was an extract of poison oak (*Rhus tox*), which homeopaths choose because in large doses it is said to produce toxic effects that mimic the symptoms of the osteoarthritic joint. Here is an account of the trial as published in *Medical News*, a weekly newspaper for doctors, designed to keep them abreast of new and interesting developments in their profession.

A group of patients with osteoarthritis of the hips or knees were admitted to the study, and allocated randomly to one of three groups—placebo, fenoprofen, or *Rhus tox*.

All patients received the three treatments, each for a period of two weeks. All other treatments were stopped, but patients were allowed to take paracetamol as an "escape" analgesic.

Before, during and after the trial, all patients were assessed and asked to rate the pain and discomfort experienced. An overall preference was sought at the end of the third treatment.

Thirty-three patients completed the trial. Two had dropped out because of an aggravation of symptoms while taking *Rhus tox*, and a further five also had exacerbation of their symptoms while on the homoeopathic remedy.

Analysis of the study results shows that there was no significant difference between the effects of *Rhus tox* and that of placebo. Fenoprofen however, produced highly significant pain relief compared with the other two.

When asked for their treatment preference, of those who could make a choice, 21 preferred fenoprofen, and five each placebo and *Rhus tox*. There were few side effects, the most common being mild gastrointestinal disturbance in patients on fenoprofen.

This is only the third controlled trial comparing homoeopathic remedies with conventional treatments, and gives little support to those homoeopaths who prescribe preparations containing *Rhus tox* as a salve for osteoarthritis.

Homeopathy as a treatment for arthritis? My verdict is "Interesting, but so far the merits are not proven." But again, if you do want to try homeopathy, do not waste time and energy by consulting anyone other than a qualified practitioner. Do not be deterred by the accusation that homeopathy is unscientific "placebo" medicine, or that it produces its effects by introducing elements of a personal character into the therapeutic process, such as the fact that homeopathic doctors usually spend more time than conventional doctors on establishing symptoms and tailoring remedies. If you appear to get relief at the hands of a homeopathic doctor whose remedies contain no dangers, then yours not to reason why. As one commentator puts it, "If homeopathy is to survive in a hostile economic and professional climate, it will have to prove its worth." And the best judge of that worth is the sufferer.

HYDROTHERAPY

Nature cures of various kinds are often tried by rheumatoid arthritis sufferers. Particularly the use of water—*hydrotherapy*—is popular, either as baths or taken internally. "Taking the waters" indeed has a long history, and can take the form of swallowing water as medicine, wrapping swollen joints in compresses, using steam inhalators, or taking baths in Epsom salts. The ancient Romans were abundantly keen on baths, and today many people still make their way to health spas in various parts of the world. Variants on the natural spa are "health hydros," seawater booths (hot or cold) called thalassotherapy, and Turkish and sauna baths.

Personally, I love to take a sauna or swim in the sea or visit charming towns such as Bath, but I find the therapeutic advantages of such activities distinctly limited so far as my RA is concerned. Sometimes a warm bath or a cool swim will certainly ease an aching ankle or finger joint, but the relief is temporary. On the other hand, I certainly feel fresher and in better tone after splashing about in water, so to that extent I suppose I am, minimally, an advocate of nature cures.

MANIPULATION AND MOVEMENT THERAPIES

When performed by a skilled individual, manipulative therapies such as massage can bring a terrific sense of well-being, and sometimes temporary relief from joint pains. Back sufferers especially seem to gravitate toward manipulation for such ailments as fibrositis and sciatica. Again, if you want to try this approach to helping with your arthritis, by all means do so. Bear in mind that manipulatory techniques take a variety of forms: Rolfing, or Structural Integration, is one that has had a lot of attention in recent years (though it dates back a few decades, in fact), as has the so-called Alexander principle for correcting postural defects. Less well known is the Feldenkrais technique for body movement and retraining, a system which has aims similar to those of the exercise and movement therapies such as yoga, t'ai chi, aikido, and dance therapy.

With yoga and the like there is, of course, a dimension beyond the purely physical. These are therapies that are calculated not simply to help you shrug off aches and pains but to train the mind and the spirit to work in harmony with the body. According to Brian Inglis and Ruth West in their comprehensive compendium of unorthodox therapies *The Alternative Health Guide*, such therapies do seem to have achieved "remarkable results" with arthritis patients, so I see no reason why one should not give them a try. But again, carefully, under expert supervision, and if you can, in a reasonably open frame of mind, neither expecting too much nor determined to prove that you will achieve little.

PSYCHOLOGICAL THERAPIES

Moving, as it were, a little farther out, there are also alternative therapies of a psychological or even psychical nature. *Hypnosis*, in particular, seems to be getting increasingly "respectable" among medical men, and here again we have a technique with a long history, especially for treating pain. This alone might make it worth exploring for your arthritis, but especially if your attacks have what is called an emotional overlay—that is, they seem to be linked to periods in your life of excessive stress or emotional strain. (I will return to this theme in the next chapter, where you will see how in my case there very definitely was a psychosomatic connection.)

There are also self-help psychological therapies: autosuggestion, Silva Mind Control, and one very interesting technique called autogenic training, a technique whereby one learns to de-stress the body through relaxation, which I have seen demonstrated and which certainly seems to work powerfully on one's stress reactions. It is not unlike meditation in its effects, or the biofeedback technique, both of which can help to strip away that emotional overlay to your disease. No one will, or rather should, promise that these techniques will directly affect the progress of your arthritis. But they can generally put you in a better, more relaxed frame of mind, more able to meet the world and perhaps better equipped to handle your own pain.

You may even try psychic healing, the "laying on of hands," which, though only offering temporary relief (if any relief at all), may give you a small but much needed psychological boost by introducing a shaft of sunlight into otherwise gloomy thoughts.

MUSSEL EXTRACT

On one occasion, an Australian friend told me about an intriguing substance that was causing a stir among rheumatologists who appeared to be in something of a quandary over its alleged properties. The preparation in question was an extract from the green-lipped mussel, a species found around the shores of New Zealand, which it was claimed had anti-inflammatory properties. At first this was only a tentative suggestion, but then a British research team in Scotland tested the extract on a group of patients with classical RA symptoms and osteoarthritis. Up to that time they had all been taking some form of NSAID. At the end of the test, the researchers claimed in *The Practitioner* (1982), a medical journal, that "the extract of the green lipped mussel, *Perna canaliculus*, is an effective supplement or possible alternative to orthodox therapy in the treatment of both rheumatoid arthritis and osteoarthritis. It reduces the amount of pain and stiffness, improves the patient's ability to cope with life, and apparently enhances general health. Added to these benefits is the low incidence of side effects. It would therefore seem that this substance could be of considerable value to patients suffering from these two chronic and disabling conditions."

Other researchers argued with these results, whereupon there was a rejoinder, and a minor controversy arose. Meanwhile, a biochemist at the Royal Melbourne Institute of Technology, Dr. Paul Gregory, was carrying out his experiments. He found that the green-lipped mussel worked well as an anti-inflammatory agent in the laboratory even though he did not altogether endorse the enthusiastic results of the Glasgow trials. Other researchers have followed up his work—using, incidentally, laboratory rats on which to test for anti-inflammatory properties—and supported his findings. I managed to acquire some of the mussel extract, and it has certainly helped me, so at the moment I am continuing to use it.

CELLULAR THERAPY

Another alternative that I am pursuing is a technique called cellular therapy which has interested me for some years. I went to a clinic in Switzerland—La Prairie, founded by an Austrian, Dr. Niehans—where they harvest fresh living cells from fetal lambs. They collect cells from all the organs separately, the kidney, liver and so on, and then they inject these cells into the patient by muscular injection. They claim that these will regenerate degenerated areas: the liver cells going to the liver, kidney cells to the kidneys, and so on. There is actually a migration of the cells to these areas. At least, that is what is claimed. I don't believe it is that way, but the point is that this clinic and others like it have been going for fifty years, and I am a great believer in the motto that you can't fool all of the people all of the time. Maybe it's psychology, maybe it's not. But people pay a lot of money to go there, and they return to the clinic, so they must find some benefit. Therefore I cannot, like many doctors, say that cellular therapy is so much rubbish, because people *do* feel better. I went there because they said that one of the conditions that they can help is arthritis. I had one course of treatment and thought at the beginning that I felt better. Then the arthritis started up again, and I went back and had another course of treatment. Now I still have arthritis, but can I fairly say that the therapy was no help at all? I have no "control" to measure myself against. What would have happened to Christiaan Barnard if he had not had that cellular therapy? Would he already today be in a wheelchair? It is difficult to say. It may have helped, though it didn't cure it, that's for sure.

Nevertheless, cellular therapy is worth investigating on a very scientific basis, and that is what I am involved in now. Can we prove beyond a shadow of a doubt that the damaged cell can regenerate or that aging cells will degenerate more slowly in the presence of fresh fetal lamb cells or components of it? If cellular therapy does work, it probably does so through some regeneration of the genetic information of a cell. You see, the aging and degenerative condition of a cell are caused by the fact that the genetic information gets mixed up and it cannot express itself properly. We know that the genetic information of a cell can be reprogrammed by the addition of genetic information (which is what probably happens when a virus invades a cell or a tumor forms). Now, cancer cells behave quite differently from normal cells in that they become immortal. Cervical cancer cells, for instance, have been growing now for I don't know how many years in laboratories where a normal cell would have died off. So perhaps cellular therapy is a means of modifying the dying-off part of a cell's genetic information store. It is, as I say, worth investigating.

The thing to remember with all of these alternative therapies is that they can only be undertaken on a "try it and see" basis. You could dabble with five, ten, even twenty methods and get no results worth writing home about, but with the twenty-first find something that seems to help a little. This might seem a strange thing for me, a doctor, to recommend, but I believe in preaching what I practice. When you have years of pain and anguish, you will try anything, within the bounds of safety. I make no bones about admitting to sampling homemade pure honey, ginseng root, and even royal jelly (the substance fed to the queen bee by her zealous workers) in the hope (vain, in this case) of alleviating matters.

ARTHRITIS AND STRESS:
A PERSONAL DIMENSION 9

This has been the most painful chapter for me to set down on paper, because it is here that I discuss aspects of my arthritis that touch on some of the more sensitive areas of my life. To be honest, I thought more than twice about doing so, but concluded that if I were to censor myself, I would be giving you an incomplete understanding of my arthritis. And hence I would have missed an opportunity to give you, perhaps, an insight into yours.

First a little autobiography, starting with a love affair. After the first transplant operations, I became famous, an internationally known celebrity invited to appear here, go there, and generally have a good time. Which I did. Life was extremely hectic, what with shouldering my professional responsibilities at the hospital and meeting my social commitments outside, so much so that you would think that this would aggravate my by then established arthritis. But curiously enough, it did not. For a while I actually improved. Then I met Barbara, and my RA virtually disappeared altogether. She was young and beautiful, and we fell in love. The affair culminated in divorce from my first wife and marriage to Barbara. The effect on my arthritis, among other things, was dramatic. I cannot offer you any "scientific" explanation, but I can say that meeting Barbara produced a degree of satisfaction in my life that may have put my body in better tune. Certainly for several years after the wedding I virtually ceased to be an RA sufferer.

After a while, though, the attacks began to reestablish themselves, especially at times of stress—and this pattern has frequently repeated itself. There is no doubt that in my case arthritis is brought on both by emotional and physical stress. For example, I found that the evening or morning after a difficult operation in which I had to use my hands in awkward positions, there would be an exacerbation of the arthritis in my fingers. Similarly, whenever I was under above-average emotional stress, the arthritis would light up. I don't know whether I was emotionally more

115

settled during the early period of marriage to Barbara (although physically I was very active), but in those days I used to joke that the cure for arthritis was to marry a young woman. I suppose I was so busy loving her that I forgot about the pains in my body. But that was only in the early days.

Anyway, the attacks seemed to come and go, often as a result of various stresses. Then came the bombshell. Barbara came to me one day saying she wanted a divorce. She had met a younger, more active man who, she said, could give her the sort of life that I could not. "What's wrong with our life?" I asked. And then it came out that arthritis had played a major part in the breakdown of the marriage. Barbara was very active, and although she tolerated the fact that sometimes I was inactive as a result of arthritis, after we divorced she told friends and newspaper reporters that I used to sleep on Saturday afternoons and that I never used to play with the children or go out to the beach with her. Well, that was all true, but not because I didn't want to; it was simply too painful for me. For example, I could not play cricket with my children without tremendous pain in my hands or wrists. And I slept often during the weekends because I was exhausted by the inflammatory process that was burning in my body all the time—the constant pain. Somehow Barbara could never accept the fact that I had a physical disability and that I could not be the active man that she thought I should be. Her younger man was more active and could take my family out on buggy rides on the beach and all that sort of stuff. So Barbara thought, "Well, this is the life that I am missing." Hence our marital breakdown.

I had an extreme emotional reaction to the divorce. I felt that life was ended for me. I was terribly jealous because Barbara was going out with someone thirty years younger than I. (In fact, he is even much younger than she.) Moreover, Barbara seemed to rub it in by telling me how great this guy was, what a beautiful body he had, and all that sort of thing. The result was that I eventually felt that I was hopeless, physically, emotionally, sexually.

Previously, I had always said that I have no inferiority complex (I don't have a superiority complex either, although I am a little vain). I had also never been jealous before in my life. If my wife doesn't love me, I thought, then she must do what she wants to do. Then I always had a tremendous ambition and drive. If I want something I get it, and I will drive for it as hard as I can. Well, virtually overnight all those qualities disappeared. I had no confidence, I had no desire to live, I contemplated suicide many times. And at those times I frequently blamed arthritis for my predicament.

I honestly feel that I would have won Barbara back if it was not for my arthritis. I just couldn't do what she wanted me to do. If I had performed physically and sexually as well as this younger guy, she would have come back to me—or so I believed at the time. I kept on saying to her, "If I didn't have the arthritis, I would be such a different man." But she made no reply. She was not prepared to display the patience and understanding that I needed at that particular moment. The divorce was right. She was correct in divorcing me because I just didn't come up to her standards anymore.

So there I was, an arthritic who blamed the loss of his wife on his disease and then found, to add injury to insult, that the marital breakdown was actually aggravating the arthritis. A truly vicious circle.

Then there were other gloomy thoughts that tortured me. I was driven to realize that I was getting older. If, as a young person, you have something good and you lose it, you feel you have time to get something good back. But when you are old, you feel that if you lose something good, you simply haven't any more time to get it back. So the sense of loss is much greater. On top of it, you still have a crippling disease that makes it even tougher to think you have lost something you cannot get back. It was almost an overwhelming burden. I lost my wife and family, my house and home, and all the things that I loved so much. In the past, I had always been able somehow to sling off setbacks by work. Successful surgery can be wonderfully restoring to the spirit. But now, with arthritis, and *anno domini* threatening, there seemed no such escape route.

I know I am not the first person to feel that time is passing me by. But in the context of all that had happened to me, I suddenly almost changed personality, with arthritis playing an increasingly prominent role. Take lecturing. Before the divorce, lecturing to any kind of audience never worried me at all. In fact, I enjoyed it immensely. I would go to a lecture virtually unprepared, and the words would tumble out as I talked. But now as I get older, I get more tense about having to lecture, and I prepare myself for it. If your reputation is as a good lecturer, then you have got to be good. Now, to make this even worse, I find that after a lecture I have a flare-up of arthritis.

I have dwelt on these unfortunate episodes in my life for one reason. It seems to me, as I look back on my marriages and divorces, the happy times and the bleak phases, that there is a strong link between arthritis—an undeniable physical disease—and emotional stress. And this is a connection that I feel any sufferer should explore fully in his or her own life.

What do I mean by stress? Not necessarily divorce or responsibilities in your job. Anyone can become stressed whatever he does and at any stage in life. The strange, and often overlooked, fact is that this ubiquitous phenomenon can actually drive us into illness.

As a heart surgeon, I know that stress plays a great part in cardiac disease of one sort or another—and remember that this is the Western world's top killer disease, far above cancer. Heart attacks used to be

SOCIAL READJUSTMENT RATING SCALE

EVENT	LIFE CRISES UNIT SCORE
Death of wife or husband	100
Divorce	73
Marital separation	65
Jail term	63
Death of close family member	63
Personal injury or illness	53
Marriage	50
Getting the sack from work	47
Marital reconciliation	45
Retirement	45
Change in health of family member	41
Pregnancy	40
Sexual problems	39
Addition of new family member	39
Major business problems	39
Change in financial state	38
Death of close friend	37
Change to different kind of work	36
Change in living arrangements with wife/husband	35
Taking on a large mortgage	31
Foreclosure of mortgage or loan	30
Change in responsibilities at work	29
Son or daughter leaving home	29
Trouble with in-laws	29
Outstanding personal achievement	28
Wife starts/stops work	26
Starting or leaving school	26
Change in living conditions	25
Revision of personal habits	24
Trouble with the boss	23
Change in working hours or conditions	20
Change in residence	20
Change of school	20
Change in recreation	19
Change in church activities	19
Change in social activity	18
Taking on a bank loan or HP debt	17
Change in sleeping habits	16
Change in number of family reunions	15
Change in eating habits	15
Vacation	13
Christmas	12
Minor violations of the law	11

SOURCE: R. H. Rahe, 1969, in *Psychotropic Drug Response—Advances in Prediction*. Editors P. R. A. May and J. R. Wittenborn, Illinois: p. 97.

blamed on our dietary habits, especially on high-cholesterol foods, and on our sedentary lifestyle, until it began to be realized that there was a third major component in the form of the stresses and strains we accumulate every day of our lives. These can take us to a state of exhaustion, then tip us over into complete physical breakdown, where the heart muscle finally gives way.

But it is not only heart disease that results from the stresses we impose on ourselves. Doctors have established a long list of disorders in which stress is a definite contributory factor. They range from insomnia to backache, from high blood pressure to arthritis.

The circumstances that produce stress-related illnesses are many and varied. Two researchers, Thomas H. Holmes and Richard H. Rahe, looked at the events which require people to make readjustments of one sort or another—both major ones, such as marital breakdown, and relatively minor ones, such as taking out a bank loan—and gave them a score. They found that anyone who totaled over 300 points in a year had an 80 percent chance of succumbing to illness; 150 to 300 points gave you a 50 percent chance. Here is their table in full.

My own mess of potage when Barbara and I divorced quickly knocked my score above the 300 mark. In fact, I probably could tick off half the items in this extensive list. So it would hardly be surprising, if Holmes and Rahe are correct in their basic assumptions about life events and illness, that my arthritic symptoms were aggravated. And I would not be the only arthritic to have suffered in this way. A London psychiatrist, Hugh Baker, studied a group of women RA sufferers and found that there was a high incidence of emotionally stressful events in the period before the onset of RA. And by "stressful" Dr. Baker meant such circumstances as being the wife of a man whose company went bankrupt, leaving him unemployed, or a woman whose partner moved out after a seven-year liaison and married someone else.

However, being in a potentially stressful situation is not necessarily going to make you ill. A lot depends on your personality. Two American doctors, Meyer Friedman and Roy Rosenman, have found that a certain type of personality, called Type A, is definitely more prone to heart disease than Type B, which has the opposite qualities. Type As are driving, ambitious, even obsessive types (of which I am undoubtedly a good example), while Type Bs are laid back, unhurried, and easygoing. Have a look at the following list of Type A characteristics to see where you fit into the scheme of things. If you can check off most of these, then your arthritis could be exacerbated by your reaction to events.

TYPE A PEOPLE . . .

> Are easily irritated
> Feel guilty when relaxing

Show impatience with people
Take on excessive responsibilities
Try to master uncontrollable situations
Get upset when things go wrong
Have difficulty confiding in people
Have trouble solving family problems
Have a severe sense of time urgency
Try to work on two or more projects at once
Neglect all aspects of personal life in favor of work
Sacrifice leisure time
Eat, move, and work rapidly
Talk fast and explosively

Now, you may be getting really worried by all this, saying to yourself, "Well, I *am* a Type A and my life has been full of changes, forcing me to readjust lately, so my arthritis will certainly get worse." But this ain't necessarily so. For one thing, there is a difference between being susceptible to disease and actually succumbing to illness. Some of the most placid and easygoing people you could meet are the Afrikaaners of South Africa, especially the farmers; yet this classic Type B is the one who has the highest incidence of coronary heart disease in the world today. I never find it at all helpful to ask a patient who comes to me with heart disease, "Are you an excitable person?" You find coronary heart disease among people who are working hard and have responsibility in life, but you also find it in people who are completely the opposite. You find that with those who work hard and have responsible positions, there are other factors. It is like the study which showed that the bus driver is more prone to coronary heart disease than the bus conductor. It was said that this was because the driver is under more stress. On the other hand, the bus driver sits on his bum all day and the conductor runs up and down. It is difficult to get a clear-cut view.

What I am sure of, though, is that any arthritic should try to reduce stress in his or her life as much as possible by finding ways of counteracting some of the inevitable ups and downs. These can take many forms. There are times when you feel hysterically overworked when you need to bring yourself up with a jolt by some kind of emergency "red light" procedure. A simple routine is advocated by Jane Madders, a specialist in antistress relaxation techniques, who has an easily remembered four-point strategy to follow when you are really getting worked up by circumstances.

1. Say "Stop" to yourself.

2. Breathe in deeply and breathe out slowly. As you do so, drop your shoulders and relax your hands.

3. Breathe in deeply again, and as you breathe out, make sure your teeth aren't clenched tightly together.

4. Take two small, quiet breaths.

Mostly, though, we need to develop techniques to practice regularly to *prevent* the stresses building up. Here I recommend you do two things.

First, explore the local opportunities for exercise, relaxation, yoga, meditation, or similar de-stressing techniques such as autogenic or bio-feedback training. Find groups which you can attend regularly, and try out various relaxation methods until you hit on one that suits you and which you can easily practice regularly at home.

Second, follow a basic, sensible recipe for keeping healthy and able to cope with everyday stresses. Here's a simple one advocated in an excellent television series produced in Britain by Thames Television called *How to Last a Lifetime*.

- Avoid serious fatigue. If this should happen, take *immediate* steps to overcome it.
- Keep a balance between rest and activity.
- Ensure enough *good-quality* sleep.
- Plan a realistic program of activities that gives plenty of time to achieve deadlines, with realistic targets that can be confidently reached.
- Try to keep some energy always in reserve.
- When demands get too much, learn to say no to yourself or others.
- Learn relaxation skills and practice them as often as possible, particularly in situations that tend to produce tension.
- Recognize your own personal limitations, and have the willpower to keep within them.

These basic precepts can be extended to your workplace. Take, for example, the planning of activities to keep within the bounds of the realistic. Time management, whereby you schedule your day's activities carefully, set priorities, and concentrate on one task at a time, should be in the mind of anyone with a busy-busy occupation. So, too, should delegating responsibilities, accepting your limitations, and learning from mistakes rather than criticizing yourself for them. All this can reduce job stress by a considerable amount.

However hard one tries to prevent or cope with stress, there will be times when you do not succeed. I found this during my divorce from Barbara, when my feet or hand joints would flare up with clockwork regularity whenever things became acrimonious between us. At times like this I felt a two-time loser: unhappy emotionally *and* with an incurable disease. And yet I tried to carry on, to fight my way through it. It is so tempting to blame my arthritis for everything that went wrong and get it out of all proportion. Yet everything I have ever achieved in life that is worth something has been achieved in the presence of and despite RA. An illness of itself does not ruin your life if you refuse to let it.

History is full of great individuals who had "something wrong" with them. To name just a few: Beethoven, deafness; Van Gogh, psychiatric disorder; Franklin Delano Roosevelt, polio; guitarist Django Reinhart, missing fingers. Not only did people like this not lie down and succumb, but, it is sometimes argued, the very fact that they were ill spurred them on to greater heights.

It all depends on how one views one's particular problem. As far as heart disease is concerned, people respond with various reactions. Some accept the fact that they have it, especially after a heart attack, and they adjust themselves to such an extent that they live under the restraints that are necessary. Others don't accept it and become hypochondriacs. There's a great variation to the behavior of people afflicted by illnesses. Some bear the cross with great intelligence and tolerance, and others find it very difficult to have these disabilities. And this goes just as much for arthritis as for any other condition.

It takes effort. Lord, it takes effort to force yourself every day to think positively about a disease that may be progressively restricting your movement and reducing you to tears of pain. But you can make the effort a little less burdensome, perhaps, by thinking about some of the ideas I have been discussing in this chapter:

1. Avoiding stressful situations
2. Modifying your attitudes toward those you cannot avoid
3. Equipping yourself with some simple antistress techniques
4. Trying not to feel sorry for yourself

Actually if you throw yourself wholeheartedly into 1, 2 and 3, number 4 will take care of itself.

DIET AND EXERCISE 10

These exercises have been adapted by kind permission of the authors and publishers from the following sources: *The Sunday Times New Book of Body Maintenance* (Eds. O. Gillie, C. Haddon and D. Mercer/Michael Joseph, 1982); *Caring for the Elderly* (S. Hooker/ Routledge & Kegan Paul, 1976); *Overcoming Arthritis* (F.D. Hart/Martin Dunitz, 1981).

Sooner or later every arthritic will ask the doctor whether there is any way to improve the condition by dietary means. A logical question, of course, in that our bodies are biochemical factories fueled by our food intake. Thus the "wrong" sort of food could arguably upset the running of the bodily machinery, as the wrong mixture of gas and air in the carburetor of your car will cause the engine to misfire and even cut out altogether. "You are," after all, "what you eat."

As a doctor whose career has been dedicated to helping people with heart disease, I more than most was certainly tempted to think that my RA might have been prevented—and could be alleviated—by reworking my eating habits. For heart disease, as I have mentioned, is undeniably associated to some extent with dietary factors: people who eat large amounts of fatty foods, especially animal fats, accumulate cholesterol-rich deposits in the walls of the arteries supplying the heart muscle, which literally clog up the flow of blood. If you add to that the fact that many people in the comparatively well-heeled Western world are walking around with too much weight on their frames, you can see that an excess of food of the wrong sort has a more or less direct deleterious effect on the cardiac system. Clogged up and overworked, it will collapse under the tremendous demands imposed on it.

Can anything like this be said of arthritis? Does any sort of food initiate joint disease or aggravate it in a person who is already a sufferer? Here is the view of the Arthritis Foundation (U.S.A.) in its pamphlet *Arthritis: Diet and Nutrition—Facts to Consider:* "As far as is currently known, no form of arthritis is caused by food, or by the wrong combination of foods. Eating special foods or eliminating others from your diet will not cure arthritis. Obviously, if you are poorly nourished, you won't be as healthy as you could be. That, in turn, will affect your general health and your ability to resist or endure the physical wear and tear of arthritis.

The Arthritis Foundation's unequivocal view is shared, I know, by many doctors. They, too, point out that gout is a special case because it is known that foods rich in purines such as sweetbreads, liver, kidney, and brain will tend to provoke attacks. As gout is produced by high levels of uric acid in the blood, any substance which drives up the levels can stimulate the formation of painful crystals. Alcohol is one. So, too, are certain diuretics or water pills which are taken to increase urine flow in people who retain too much fluid and salt in the body. But apart from gout, the official view seems to be that there is no point in thinking about "special" diets for arthritis.

What matters, then, is regular, balanced meals drawn from a wide range of easily available foods. These will ensure good overall health, muscle tone, and the capacity to resist the wear and tear causing degenerative joint disease.

Not everyone agrees, though, with this easy-to-follow prescription. I once went to a clinic where they eat only raw vegetables, fruits, and nuts. The doctor there had a bottle into which he poured a typical selection of supermarket-style food: a bowl of soup, then some ketchup, meat, rice, then ice cream and chocolate sauce. He then shook it up, saying, "That is how your stomach looks inside after you eat this food." He called it "putrefaction," and I was horrified by the sight.

At this clinic I was put on a very strict diet of raw stuff. No sugar, no salt. Massages every day for one hour. A colonic lavage to clear out the bowels. I followed the regime for about two weeks before leaving. It may have been psychological, but I think I felt better—not enough, though, to persuade me to stick with what was in all honesty a rather boring diet.

Another, more varied approach is that adopted by the Chinese-American doctor Collin H. Dong, who at the age of thirty-five, after practicing medicine for seven years, was afflicted with arthritis that no amount of painkillers and anti-inflammatory agents seemed to help. On top of the pains in various joints Dr. Dong also contracted severe dermatitis, his hair began to fall out, and his face puffed up to produce a pitiful sight—and all this despite the fact that he had consulted a number of prominent experts in rheumatology. Dr. Dong became interested in an idea that has grown in popularity in recent years, namely that his considerable range of symptoms might be the result of allergy to certain foods. So he set out to develop a nutritional program, specifically for arthritics, that took into account the allergy potential in many of the substances we all regularly consume without a second thought. As a result he makes some suggestions that he admits are initially difficult to accept, for old habits die hard. However, the rewards he claims are fantastically encouraging, tantamount to a "cure." Here in bald outline are his suggestions.

DO'S AND DON'TS

DO EAT OR DRINK

All seafoods
All vegetables, including avocados
Vegetable oils, particularly safflower and corn
Margarine free of milk solids
Egg whites
Honey
Nuts, sunflower seeds, soya bean products
Rice of all kinds: brown, white, wild
Bread to which nothing listed under DO NOT EAT OR DRINK has been added
Tea and coffee
Plain soda water
Parsley, onions, garlic, bay leaf, salt
Any kind of flour
Sugar

DO NOT EAT OR DRINK

Meat in any form, including broth
Fruit of any kind, including tomatoes
Dairy products, including egg yolks, milk, cheese, yogurt
Vinegar, or any other acid
Pepper (definitely)
Chocolate
Dry roasted nuts (the process involves monosodium glutamate)
Alcoholic beverages
Soft drinks (I have never found one without additives)
All additives, preservatives, chemicals, most especially monosodium glutamate. One exception to this rule is the lecithin in margarine.

PERHAPS OCCASIONALLY

Breast of chicken and chicken broth
A small amount of wine in cooking
A small drink of whisky
A small pinch of spicy seasoning such as curry powder
Noodles or spaghetti, since the amount of egg is relatively small and somewhat broken down in the cooking

EXCEPTIONS

Persons who have gout, or who have been diagnosed as having what is called gouty arthritis, will do well to avoid certain things. This sensitivity must be determined by the individual, since it varies from person to person, but in general mushrooms, asparagus, spinach, artichokes, peas, and beans are possible offenders. As for alcohol, whisky does not seem to be right for some people with gout; I would suggest vodka for their rare indulgence.

From Collin H. Dong and Jane Banks,
The Arthritic's Cookbook (Granada, 1983).

Clearly there is conflict between the sort of dietary regime advocated by Dr. Dong with his allergy therapy and the mainstream of orthodox physicians, who, except for gout, are reluctant to implicate specific foods directly in the onset or aggravation of joint problems. For my part, I tend to range myself on the side of orthodoxy. I have tried special diets by the dozen. I have investigated the merits of high-fiber intake, cut out foods with chemical additives as far as possible, eaten fresh as opposed to processed meals. On no score can I say that any one food is good or bad for my RA. Diet, in my opinion, plays no role in arthritis control—except on the question of overeating. This is where I and everyone else, orthodox or not, are in agreement. Here there is one simple-to-state rule: Do not eat too much.

Obesity and arthritis simply do not mix. Look at yourself undressed, and assess the shape you see before you. Consult the table of desirable weights for a given height on page 127. Then ask yourself if you are carrying an unwanted passenger of fat around with you.

If the answer is yes, consider these implications. On average, fatter people live shorter lives, their hearts are more stressed, their joints wear more rapidly, and their everyday movements are more difficult. The fatter you are, the less exercise you want to take, which makes you fatter, which further takes away the will to exercise, and so on in a spiral into total inactivity if you are not very careful. Your painful joints are even more painful as you keep on them the unnecessary bodily loads of excess weight. At six foot one I weigh only seventy-one kilos (156 pounds), which, according to the desirable weights chart, puts me on the slim side. Personally I welcome this. If I had had to stand in the operating theater carrying a Friar Tuck paunch, I doubt very much whether my arthritic feet would have carried me through many of those longer, tricky phases of open-heart surgery.

Watch, then, what you weigh. Be honest with yourself. If you are over the reasonable limits in the danger zone of obesity, keep to a weight-control diet. By this I do not mean that you should, if you are flabby, immediately go on an all-out crash reduction jag. Many a would-be dieter has done this, then rebounded back on a food binge that has made him or her more obese than before. Reduce weight sensibly, keeping a careful eye on balance in your food intake; going easy on alcohol, especially high-calorie spirits; trying to maintain variety in the meals you eat; cutting down on obvious waistline-ruiners such as cakes, candies, fried foods, potatoes, fats, and sugars.

Remember these tips, which I find useful in my everyday eating:

- Regular small meals are better than one huge blow-out.
- Avoid "automatic" eating—that is, taking rapid, thoughtless mouthfuls. Small mouthfuls, carefully savored, usually mean fewer calories.
- Cut the appetite with warm drinks instead of food.

DESIRABLE WEIGHTS FOR GIVEN HEIGHTS, AGE 25 AND OVER[1]

	WEIGHT IN POUNDS (IN INDOOR CLOTHING) MEN		
HEIGHT (IN SHOES)[2]	SMALL FRAME	MEDIUM FRAME	LARGE FRAME
5 ft. 2 in.	112–120	118–129	126–141
5 ft. 3 in.	115–123	121–133	129–144
5 ft. 4 in.	118–126	124–136	132–148
5 ft. 5 in.	121–129	127–139	135–152
5 ft. 6 in.	124–133	130–143	138–150
5 ft. 7 in.	128–137	134–147	142–161
5 ft. 8 in.	132–141	138–153	147–166
5 ft. 9 in.	136–145	142–156	151–170
5 ft. 10 in.	140–150	146–160	155–174
5 ft. 11 in.	144–154	150–165	159–179
6 ft. 0 in.	148–158	154–170	164–184
6 ft. 1 in.	152–162	158–175	168–189
6 ft. 2 in.	156–167	162–180	173–194
6 ft. 3 in.	160–171	167–185	178–199
6 ft. 4 in.	164–175	172–190	182–204

	WOMEN		
	SMALL FRAME	MEDIUM FRAME	LARGE FRAME
4 ft. 10 in.	92–98	96–107	104–119
4 ft. 11 in.	94–101	98–110	106–122
5 ft. 0 in.	96–104	101–113	109–125
5 ft. 1 in.	99–107	104–116	112–128
5 ft. 2 in.	102–110	107–119	115–131
5 ft. 3 in.	105–113	110–122	118–134
5 ft. 4 in.	108–116	113–126	121–138
5 ft. 5 in.	111–119	116–130	125–142
5 ft. 6 in.	114–123	120–135	129–146
5 ft. 7 in.	118–127	124–139	133–150
5 ft. 8 in.	122–131	128–143	137–154
5 ft. 9 in.	126–135	132–147	141–158
5 ft. 10 in.	130–140	136–151	145–163
5 ft. 11 in.	134–144	140–155	149–168
6 ft. 0	138–148	144–159	153–174

[1] Those associated with longest life. Note that these weights are less than the average and also that desirable adult weight remains the same throughout adulthood from age 25, whereas average weights rise to a maximum at ages 50–59.

[2] 1-inch heels for men and 2-inch heels for women.

SOURCE: Joan Gomez, *How Not to Die Young* (London: Allen & Unwin, 1973).

• If you are having trouble sticking with it, team up with a friend or join a weight-watchers' organization.

Along with purely dietary measures, you should also think of reducing or maintaining your weight by regular exercise. Here I have in mind recreational or fitness exercise of one sort or another, such as taking an active part in sports. For most of us I suppose the most readily available exercise is walking, jogging (preferably on soft ground), swimming, and cycling, though there are of course literally hundreds of other enjoyable ways of keeping the body trim and burning off excess calories. The criteria to adopt are: what exercise do you genuinely like to take (no use being self-sacrificial about it) and can you take it regularly without producing pain or inflammation in the affected joints?

Apart from fitness activities, which generally make you feel better and keep you slimmer, there are a number of exercises designed to be of specific help to the arthritic. These are calculated to give the joint its natural range of movement, keeping it supple and mobile, without imposing any strains or distortions of an abnormal kind. They should be performed regularly, every day, morning and evening if possible, preferably when you are warmed up from a bath or shower. Most physiotherapists working in rheumatology departments can give you printed instructions on this kind of exercise, but you may like to know which I found most useful. If you want to attempt any but the most gentle of these, do please check with your doctor or physiotherapist that they are appropriate for you personally.

GENERAL EXERCISES

Flexibility exercises

These exercises need an upright chair. If you can't make a movement, don't. Never strain yourself.

With a scarf under the shoe, using it as a lever, gently pull each foot up several times.

For waist mobility, start with your hands on either side of the chair and swivel round.

For swollen ankles, hook or cross one leg over the other. Press toes up, down, out, in, then circle round one way and the other.

Keeping feet on the ground, lift up heels then toes. Do with each foot, then both together.

For neck flexibility, let the head sag forward (don't push), then lift it up. Let it fall to the side, then bring it up. Do this both sides.

Sit in the chair, bottom right at the back and spine touching the chair-back all the way up. Draw yourself up—chest out, head up.

UNCURLING:

This is how to do the body exercise described immediately below.

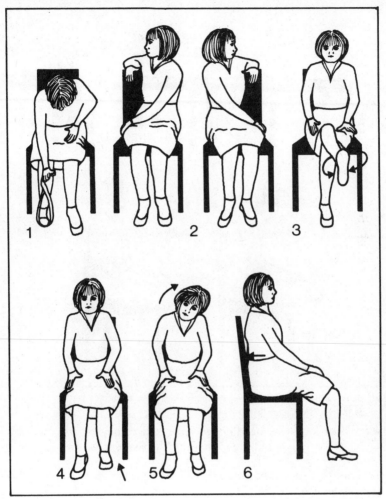

Based on illustrations from *The Sunday Times New Book of Body Maintenance* (Michael Joseph, 1982).

BODY

Sit comfortably in a chair. Drop your head forward so that it touches your chest. Then gradually lean downwards towards your knees. Straighten up again, not unwinding your head until last.

EXERCISES FOR THE SPINE

The three movements of your spine which you should practice (unless your back is too acutely painful to make it possible) are bending back-

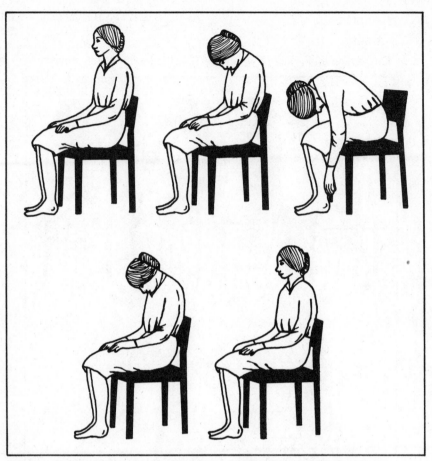

Based on illustrations appearing in *Overcoming Arthritis* by Frank Dudley Hart, published in paperback by Martin Dunitz.

wards and forwards, bending sideways and turning to left and right. These exercises will put the spine through each of those movements:

1. Stand up and bend forward toward your toes as far as you can. Then straighten up and, folding your arms across your chest, lean backwards so that you are looking towards the ceiling. Then bend forwards again. The exercise should be done as a gentle, continuous curling, starting at the base of the spine and working upward. It can also be done while lying down.
2. Stand up straight and then bend slowly sideways, running your left hand down your left thigh. Then straighten up again and do the same to the right.
3. Put your hands on your hips and rotate your spine so that, without moving your feet, you turn first to face the right and then to the left.

Exercises suitable for bronchitis, Parkinson's Disease, and 'backward tilt'. (People with 'backward tilt' should only do the forward bending exercises.)

(a) Lying as flat as possible on the bed.
  i Press the head and shoulders hard back into the bed. Relax, and repeat 10 times.
  ii Using the tummy muscles, lift the head up to look at the feet. 10 times.
(b) Sitting on an upright chair.
  i Put the head back and arch the back while taking a deep breath in. Relax and breathe out. Repeat slowly 5 times.
  ii Sitting up straight, twist the body round to look behind, keeping the seat squarely on the chair, repeat turning the other way. 5 times.
  iii Lean forward to put the head on the knees. 5 times.
     NOTE: Do not do this exercise if it causes giddiness.

EXERCISES FOR THE FEET, ANKLES, AND KNEES

FEET AND ANKLES

Exercises suitable for foot strain, swollen feet and legs, cramp, leg ulcers, and stroke.
(a) Sit with the knees crossed.
  i Pull the foot up and down from the ankle; when pushing down point the toes hard towards the floor. 20 times. Repeat with the other foot.
  ii Circle the foot round from the ankle drawing a large circle in the air with the big toe. 10 times. Repeat with the other foot.
  iii Bend the toe joints on the raised foot as far as possible up and down; then relax. 5 times. Repeat with the other foot.
(b) Sit with both feet flat on the floor, knees at a right angle.
  i Keeping the balls of the feet on the ground raise the heels as

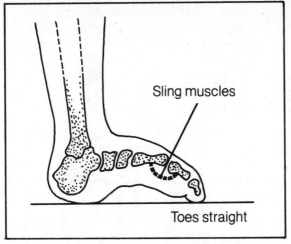

Sling muscles

Toes straight

Based on illustrations from *Caring for the Elderly* (Routledge & Kegan Paul, 1976).

high as possible; the top of the foot should be almost vertical each time. 10 times.

  ii Press the toes flat against the floor and while keeping them straight raise the ball of the foot off the ground to make a bridge. (This is a small movement but is important in re-educating the small 'sling' muscles supporting the arches of the foot.) 10 times. Repeat with the other foot.

(c) Lying on the bed with the legs raised on pillows.

  i Pull the feet up and down from the ankle, alternately in a pedalling motion. Particular care should be taken to push right down, making the calf muscles work strongly to create a pumping action which helps to drain fluid out of the feet and legs. Keep the legs up for half an hour. This exercise can also be done while sitting down during the day with feet up on a stool.

KNEES

Exercises suitable for osteoarthrosis, rheumatoid arthritis, stroke, Parkinson's Disease, fractured 'hip', unsteadiness, and knees that 'give way'.

(a) Sit with the legs out straight on a stool, or sit on the bed.

  i Brace the knees back by tightening the thigh muscles. The back of the knees should be pushed against the stool or bed. Keep them tight for a minute, then relax. Tighten really hard and relax. 20 times with each leg.

  ii Brace the knees back as before, and when the muscles are really tight lift one leg off the stool keeping the whole leg quite straight. It is only necessary to lift about a foot off the stool before putting it slowly down. The whole point of the exercise is lost if the knee is allowed to bend at any point. 10 times with each leg, increasing the number as the strength grows.

  iii Bend the knees alternately to bring the heel as close to the buttock as possible. 10 times with each leg.

Exercise bicycles for use indoors are useful for maintaining knee movements and building up muscle tone in the legs. However, even without

Based on illustrations from *Caring for the Elderly* (Routledge & Kegan Paul, 1976).

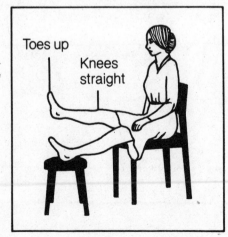

Toes up

Knees straight

such special apparatus you can benefit from lying on your back and doing cycling movements in the air for two or three minutes. Two slightly less strenuous knee exercises you can do are as follows:

1. Lie on your back and slowly bend up one knee as far as it will go, then stretch the leg out straight again. Then do the same with your other leg and repeat the exercise several times.
2. Lie straight with your feet pointing upwards. Slowly lift one leg (not necessarily very high, but just so that it is not touching the bed) keeping your knee straight and your thigh muscles braced. Lower it again slowly until the calf touches the bed and then relax. Again, do the exercise with each leg in turn.

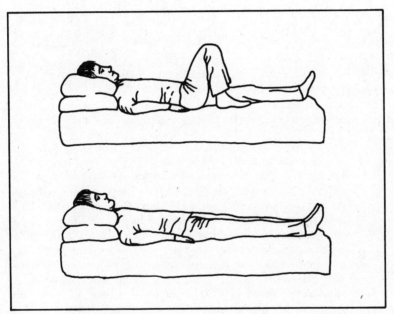

Based on illustrations appearing in *Overcoming Arthritis* by Frank Dudley Hart, published in paperback by Martin Dunitz.

EXERCISES FOR THE HIPS

Exercises suitable for arthritis of the hips, fractured 'hip', Parkinson's Disease, stroke.

(a) Lying on your side on the bed.
    i With the uppermost leg straight lift it up in the air about a foot, and bring it *slowly* down onto the other. 10 times. Turn over and repeat with the other leg.
(b) Sitting up on the bed.
    i Bend one knee onto the chest. If necessary pull the hands round the knee and give a sustained pull. 5 times with each leg.

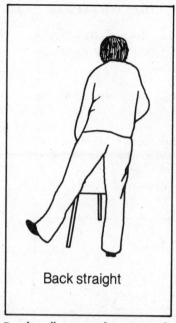

Back straight

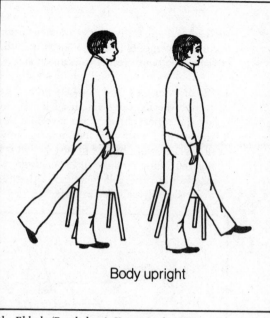

Body upright

Based on illustrations from *Caring for the Elderly* (Routledge & Kegan Paul, 1976).

(c) Standing, holding on to the back of a chair.
  i Facing the chair, swing the affected leg sideways as far as possible. A special effort must be made to keep the supporting leg straight, and the body upright. It is easy to allow the whole body to lean away from the affected leg, which results in the movement taking place in the back and good hip, while the other does not move at all. 10 times.
  ii Standing sideways to the chair, swing the affected leg forwards and backwards, again, keeping the body upright to avoid movement in the wrong place. The backward movement is very important and helps to maintain a normal gait. 10 times.
(d) Sitting on an upright chair.
  i Bend forward to put the head as near the knees as possible. 10 times.
  NOTE: Do not do this exercise if it causes giddiness.

The important thing with the hip is to rotate the joint so that the capsule around it does not contract or 'knit up'. A good exercise to help this is to lie on your back and slowly bend up both your legs. Separate your knees as wide apart as you can but keeping your heels together, and then close them back together again. Finally stretch out first one leg and then the other so that you are lying down straight as you were at the beginning.

Another hip exercise also begins in this position, lying on your back with your legs outstretched. One leg at a time, and keeping your knees straight, you lift your leg just clear of the bed, move it slowly out to the

134

side as far as you can and then return it to its original position. Do these exercises several times until the joints begin to feel freer.

If your hips are stiff these movements will of course be restricted, but practicing regularly will produce results as your range of movement gradually gets wider and less painful.

LOOSENING YOUR HIPS:

1. Bring your knees up . . .
2. and out . . .
3. then together again.
4. Straighten each leg in turn.

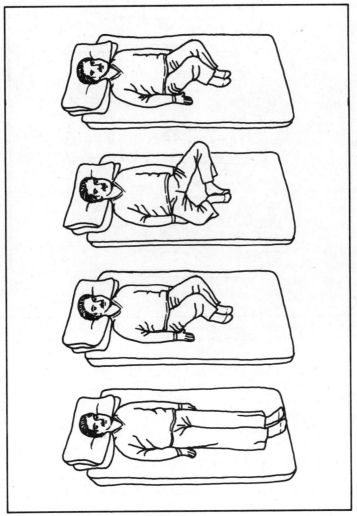

Based on illustrations appearing in *Overcoming Arthritis* by Frank Dudley Hart, published in paperback by Martin Dunitz.

SCISSORS EXERCISE:

1. Lie flat.

2. Lift your leg up off the bed . . .

3. and take it out to the side. Then repeat the exercise with the other leg.

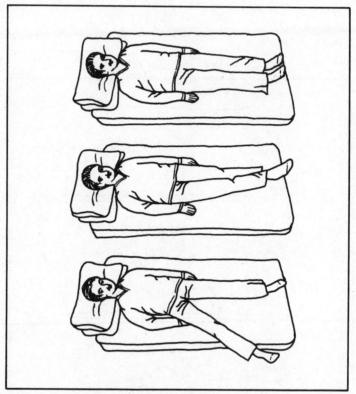

Based on illustations appearing in *Overcoming Arthritis* by Frank Dudley Hart, published in paperback by Martin Dunitz.

EXERCISES FOR THE SHOULDERS AND NECK

SHOULDERS

Exercises suitable for stroke, fractured upper arm, rheumatoid arthritis, and arthritis of the shoulder joint. The last three conditions should not be exercised in the very acute stage.

(a) Sitting on an upright chair which has no arms.
  i Let the arm hang down by the side and swing it forwards and backwards in a pendular movement. 5 times to begin with, increasing to 20 times.
  ii With the arm hanging as before swing it away from the side. 5 times increasing daily to 20 times.

iii   Supporting the hand and wrist, raise the elbow away from the side. 5 times increasing daily to 20 times.

iv   With the hand on the lap try to lift it up to the mouth as if eating. 10 times.

v   Lift the arm up to place the hand behind the neck as if combing the back of the hair. 5 times.

vi   Place the hand behind the back and try to reach up to the shoulder blades. 5 times.

vii   Lift the arm right up above the head as if reaching a shelf. If this is difficult at first, help it a little by supporting the wrist with the good hand. This exercise is particularly important in preventing a painful shoulder in people who have had a stroke.

viii   Lift and circle the shoulders, first one way and then the other, trying for maximum mobility. 5 times each way.

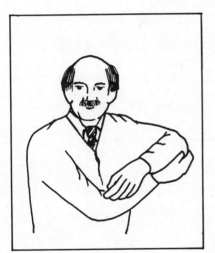 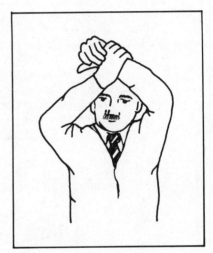

Based on illustrations from *Caring for the Elderly* (Routledge & Kegan Paul, 1976).

NECK

Exercises suitable for osteoarthrosis, Parkinson's Disease, and bronchitis.

(a)   Sitting on an upright chair.

i   Move the head forwards and back, the backward movement being very important, particularly for those with Parkinson's Disease. 5 times slowly.

ii   Circle the head round making it go as far as possible in each direction. 5 times, slowly.

NOTE: Exercises for the neck can make some people giddy and should be performed very slowly. If any giddiness occurs they should be discontinued.

EXERCISES FOR THE ELBOWS, WRIST, AND HANDS

Exercises suitable for fractured wrist, osteo- and rheumatoid arthritis of the hands, and stroke.

(a) Sitting in a chair.
   i   Make a fist with the fingers, and then straighten them out as far as possible. Repeat with each hand. 20 times.
   ii With the fingers straight spread them out to make wide spaces between each. 20 times.
   iii With the palm uppermost, take the thumb across to the tip of the little finger, run the thumb down to the base. Repeat with each other finger. 5 times.
   iv Circle the thumb round in large rings. 10 times.
   v   Holding the elbow in to the side move the hand up and down from the wrist. 10 times.
   vi Keeping the elbow in, circle the hand round in large circles. Unless the elbow is kept in, the movement occurs at the shoulder and not the wrist. 10 times.
   vii Holding a stick about the width of a walking stick, grip it tightly, and relax the grip. 10 times. Using a cloth or piece of washing wring the water out getting it as dry as possible. Doing some hand washing is excellent exercise after the plaster is taken off after a fractured wrist, but heavy articles such as towels should be avoided for a while.

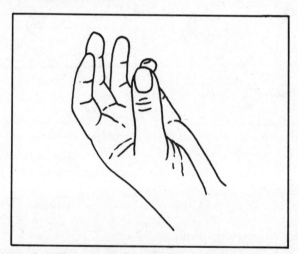

Based on illustrations from *Caring for the Elderly* (Routledge & Kegan Paul, 1976).

It is best to do these exercises with one arm at a time so that you can concentrate on that one, otherwise you will tend to find that whichever arm is the stronger ends up doing the most work.

The elbow's main movement is that of bending and stretching, so exercising this is simply a matter of sitting comfortably and bending and straightening your arm slowly as far as it will go in each direction.

The best wrist exercise is to rotate each wrist right round. Sit with your elbows tucked in to your sides and move each hand in a complete circle, first in one direction and then in the other.

To exercise your hands as fully as possible you should try regularly squeezing them into a tight fist and then slowly stretching out your fingers as wide as possible, separating them from each other and then bringing them together again.

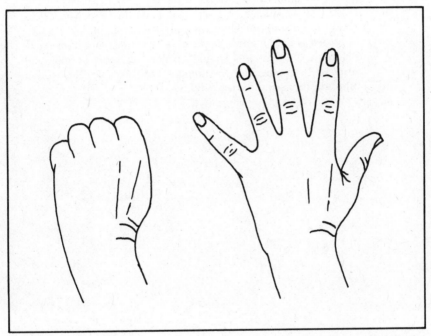

Based on illustrations appearing in *Overcoming Arthritis* by Frank Dudley Hart, published in paperback by Martin Dunitz.

One exercise which, if you can complete it, will show that most of the joints in your arm are supple is the following. You begin by raising your arms above your head with the hands pressed flat against each other, palm to palm. Then, keeping the hands pressed together, you gradually bend your elbows and bring your hands down to your chest until your fingers are just below your chin. Then rotate your wrists forward until your fingers are pointing downward. This is, of course, an ambitious exercise which involves a number of different movements on each joint and will only be possible for people whose arms and shoulders are very mobile.

BREATHING EXERCISES

Exercises suitable for all old people but particularly those with bronchitis, Parkinson's Disease, rheumatoid arthritis, circulatory disturbances and coldness of the hands and feet, and the bedfast.

(a) Sitting in a comfortable chair or half lying on the bed. The back should be supported in a straight position.

   i With the hands on the lower ribs push the ribs *out* as the breath is drawn *in*. Breathe out fully but without force. 5 times.

   ii With the hands on the stomach between the ribs, push the stomach *out* as the breath is drawn *in*. Relax and breathe out fully, letting the stomach sink down. 5 times.

NOTE: All breathing exercises should be done slowly. Taking deep breaths too quickly causes giddiness. The number I have indicated is only a guide as people's breathing capacities are so different; the exercises should be done in short periods with rests in between. The breathing should also be practiced in other positions and during activity.

LOOKING AHEAD: ARTHRITIS RESEARCH 11

So often medical research is misunderstood. And in two quite opposite ways. Some people think that the life of a research scientist is extraordinarily dry and dull: hours on end spent poring over incomprehensible (to the outsider) computer printouts or setting up tedious experiments that lead nowhere, except perhaps to other, similar experiments. For others, to be a researcher is to be a real-life equivalent of a TV soap-opera character, making key discoveries in a glamorous setting of bubbling test tubes and sizzlingly attractive lab assistants. Just one small step away from a cure for this or a wondrous treatment for that. A kind of *Dallas* played out in white coats with the smell of a Bunsen burner replacing that of expensive Havana cigars.

In truth, research is neither glamorous nor dull. It has, like any job, its routine side and from time to time its monotony. And it has its moments of sheer joy, when results come out according to expectations or, even more exciting, when the data unexpectedly yield an insight that then leads perhaps to a major accomplishment. As someone who has done a share of research, I reckon that to do it successfully you need a dogged sort of curiosity, a tireless approach to problems, however tiny, that drives you to worry at them until they either yield to a solution or reveal themselves as issues that are simply not worth pursuing. Good researchers, of course, need good brains. But they also need a streak of stubbornness in their makeup that makes them hang on, limpetlike, to their objectives in the face of fatigue, boredom, and sometimes acute despair.

Arthritis, like many other medical conditions, clearly poses some major questions for researchers: about what causes some forms to develop; about how they can be treated; and the Holy Grail of all biomedical work, whether arthritis can ever be cured—and if so, in what direction a cure might be found. In this chapter I would like to pay tribute to the creative

141

stubbornness of arthritis researchers by pointing to a few representative examples of their current work and to what the way ahead seems to be.

First, research into the actual mechanisms of arthritis. Sometimes arthritic women who become pregnant find that their symptoms diminish or even disappear altogether, only to return after the baby is born. About 75 percent of women with RA experience this kind of improvement in pregnancy, usually toward the end of the third month and continuing for a few days or even weeks after the delivery. So obviously something about the massive changes in body chemistry occasioned by becoming pregnant is effecting a remission. Research in the United States and Britain has revealed that during pregnancy women have exceptionally high levels of a protein called pregnancy-associated globulin (PAG for short) circulating in their bloodstreams. As PAG levels rise and fall, it seems that the swelling, inflammation, and pain in the joints increase and decrease in harmony. Those women who in pregnancy show little or no detectable increase in PAG have no improvement in their RA symptoms. These seem to be the unlucky 25 percent.

Now, the interesting feature of PAG is that it is thought to be responsible in part for preventing rejection of the fetus. Remember that a fetus— being 50 percent mother and 50 percent father genetically—is a half "foreign" tissue, but it is not rejected by the mother's body as a surgical transplant might be. PAG seems to help ensure that this is so. But inflammation—the culprit in RA—is thought to be caused by the same processes as those involved in rejection. So by suppressing one, PAG may be diminishing the other. Thus, there could be a new type of anti-inflammatory drug in the offing here, one which might stimulate the body to produce its own PAG or perhaps a synthetic version of the anti-inflammatory part of the PAG molecule which could be administered directly. And such a drug might not necessarily be limited in its application to women. There is, in fact, quite a lot of research into hormones associated with pregnancy and the menopause, as well as the effects of the oral contraceptive and related matters, which ties in with the remarkable PAG finding, and I feel sure that somewhere from all this will come an important clue to the causes, prevention, and perhaps even cure of rheumatoid arthritis.

Another important field of investigation, which I touched on in an earlier chapter, is the genetic factors that predispose toward arthritis, or not as the case may be. It has been found that seven out of ten people who develop RA have in common a protein called the HLA DRW4 antigen. One theory that has been proposed is that RA might be triggered by a virus which is able to "disguise" itself so that it mimics the composition of this HLA DRW4 antigen. The body, then, instead of attacking the alien virus, accepts it into its midst, having been tricked into thinking that the virus is self, as opposed to not-self. Again, it is possible that a new treatment, based on drugs that interfere with the body's immune system, might be developed to strengthen the RA sufferer's reaction to the disease. This could even lead to developing a vaccine to protect people who are known to be most at risk to RA by virtue of their antigen makeup.

Arthritis is always turning up surprises for researchers. Take the case of a totally new type of juvenile RA discovered in the affluent community of Lyme, Connecticut. Doctors became suspicious when twelve children in that small community of five thousand people suddenly succumbed to what was diagnosed as juvenile rheumatoid arthritis. At the same time, a woman reported that she, her husband, two of their children, and their neighbors all had arthritis.

It certainly was arthritis. And it could be carried by insects, according to Dr. Allen Steere, a rheumatologist at Yale University. His suspicion was supported by the fact that the disease is prevalent in sparsely populated, heavily wooded areas, and by the fact that the disease is encountered during summer and autumn, when insects are most active. Suddenly at least one type of arthritis appears to be an insect-transmitted disease. Could there be others?

Another surprise came from an Australian researcher, Dennis Lowther, of Monash University in Melbourne, who stated that many of the analgesic drugs used to control arthritic pain and inflammation such as aspirin may actually hasten the process that has caused the symptoms to arise. Using the electron microscope, Professor Lowther found that although the connective tissue or cartilage that acts as a lubricating pad between bone joints appears smooth, it is in fact a network of protein fibers impregnated with a "molecular gel." This gel is the lubricant, renewed every eight days or so in the normal course of events. But certain anti-arthritis drugs, it is claimed, actually decrease the manufacture of replacement gel, thus increasing friction at the critical junction of the joint. Certainly I have a feeling (and it is no more than that) that since I started to take anti-inflammatory drugs I have had fewer remissions from my arthritis, as if my body were being encouraged to develop a tolerance. In other words, those drugs might be making the actual disease worse.

You can see how studying the many complexities of arthritis is akin to carrying out an involved criminological investigation: looking for culprits, reconstructing circumstances, finding evidence, and following up leads— some, of course, false. The comparison is even more pointed when you learn that one rheumatologist, Dr. Jeffrey Rosenberg of the Bone and Joint Research Unit at the London Hospital, suggested that the genetic abnormalities found in people with ankylosing spondylitis may be shown up by looking at their fingerprints! A likely story, you might say, until you consider that it is a method that appears in some measure to work. Here is an account of Rosenberg's experiment by the broadcaster John Newell.

Rosenberg selected one hundred ankylosing spondylitis patients from among those attending the London Hospital, and with the aid of Scotland Yard took their fingerprints. Then he compared these in minute detail with two sets of controls, one hundred healthy normal medical students, and one hundred healthy normal people chosen from Scotland Yard's collection of more than one million fingerprints. The second set of controls were used as a double check, a way of making sure that the first set, of medical students, really were average. Results showed that there were small but significant differences, in the prints of the little fingers.

Dr. Rosenberg emphasises that this doesn't mean that fingerprints can be used to diagnose ankylosing spondylitis or any other disease. What it *does* mean is that fingerprints can be used by research scientists as an additional clue—to discover whether genetic abnormalities or unusual gene patterns play any part in various diseases, since the results from the ankylosing spondylitis research suggest that this will be the case. (Source: BBC External Services)

Still on the fingerprint theme, a rheumatologist in Cambridge, England, Dr. Richard Salsburg, may have devised a method for measuring inflammation in joints—a difficult thing for doctors to do accurately. The test is simple and safe and involves thermography—picking out infrared radiation from an object on a special camera and displaying this on a television screen. According to Dr. Salsburg, you can take a "thermographic fingerprint" of an inflamed joint, which will give you the characteristic heat patterns of an arthritic condition. The doctor can then tell exactly how well his treatments are working—and, of course, put the claims of the pharmaceutical companies for their products into (thermographic) perspective.

At this point, it seems appropriate to look at new drug research. Here a lot of attention is, understandably, focused on that archenemy, inflammation. Inflammation appears to occur when a joint produces, or rather overproduces, the hormone prostaglandin. Aspirin will reduce inflammation by inhibiting the action of an enzyme which is responsible for making prostaglandin. So, too, will steroids, though in a different way. Steroids appear to inhibit prostaglandin production at an earlier stage, by stopping the release of the raw materials necessary to build up the hormone. The key factor in stopping this release is a protein which researchers are now trying to isolate, analyze, and perhaps synthesize. If they do, they may have made a drug with the very effective anti-inflammatory properties of steroids but without their side effects.

Another, quite different approach is to find ways to stimulate the body's immune system to counteract inflammation by improving what's called cell-mediated immunity—the capacity of defense cells (phagocytes) to destroy foreign intruders. This is a curious line of research because, as we saw earlier, RA has been treated with drugs which *suppress* the immune system with some success. Here, though, the opposite tactic is employed. The idea is to make the immune system more effective by stimulating the phagocytes. By administering a drug called Levamisole, Dr. Ted Buskisson and his colleagues at St. Bartholomew's Hospital in London have been able to improve cell-mediated immunity and lessen RA symptoms. The phagocytes are, it seems, stimulated enough to mop up the irritating compounds within the joints. Of course, early trials, though promising, are not enough. More careful work has to be carried out, especially on the long-term side effects of Levamisole, if any. But this does strike me as a very promising sort of treatment that could be the forerunner of later generations of effective drugs.

So, too, is the work carried out, so far only on experimental animals, by researchers at Aston University near Birmingham, England, who have discovered that a drug commonly used for treating leprosy, Dapsone, substantially reduces the characteristic RA symptoms of inflammation, heat, swelling, and pain—without the long-term side effects of cortisone-type compounds. The same scientists also found, in the course of other animal studies, two or three compounds which may do more than simply relieve symptoms. They seem actually to reverse cartilage degeneration in joints by blocking the action of destructive enzymes. If these compounds can be shown to be useful with humans, something of a breakthrough will be around the corner. Though not, I must stress, until much more follow-up research has been done. And that takes time.

Meanwhile, other scientists are looking at the existing drugs in an effort to find ways of delivering these more effectively. Corticosteroids are known to produce immense relief but at the expense of serious side effects. One possible way to get around this dilemma is to deliver smaller doses of steroids more accurately to the parts of the body where they are needed—which means precise targeting. One approach to this is being developed in Britain, using a most ingenious technique, described here by John Newell:

> The drug is enclosed in microscopic spherical droplets of thick oil, and a suspension of these droplets is then injected directly into the joint. The droplets are too big to leak out of the joint and, sooner or later, they are swallowed by the synovial fluid's own scavenging system, living cells called macrophages which wander about literally eating up any rubbish they find lying about and so keeping things clean. Now here's the clever bit—the macrophages are the cells which cause the pain and inflammation found in arthritis. So the drug in the liposomes [i.e., the droplets] is going to just where it will do most good, right inside the cells which need to be quietened down because they are overactive. (Source: BBC External Services)

So far these tests have only been carried out on rabbits, but even so the oil droplet or liposome technique seems to be fifty to one hundred times more effective than injections carried out in the usual way. I expect to see this homing device developed to such a level that human arthritics will enjoy its undoubted benefits.

I also find it encouraging to learn that arthritis sufferers may be able to benefit from research and treatments in other fields of medicine. It may surprise you to learn that there could be cross-fertilization between arthritis research and cancer research. A tumor will not grow without a blood supply, so drugs are being tested that will prevent the formation of blood vessels to nourish malignancies. Similarly, in OA and RA, cartilages develop a pad of tiny capillaries called a pannus all over their surface, which is followed by roughening and pitting of the cartilage—typical and hitherto irreversible signs of arthritis. Could a blood vessel inhibitor for tumors also prevent cartilage deterioration? It is an intriguing thought, as is the recent suggestion that doses of x-radiation, used to treat a form of cancer called Hodgkin's disease, may be used to treat arthritis. Some trials have been carried out already with limited success, but as the *New England Journal of Medicine* (22 Oct. 1981) commented, until the results of well-organized long-term studies of radiation therapy are in hand, "this genie should be kept in the bottle."

SOME REFLECTIONS 12

You will have realized by now that temperamentally I have never felt "suited" to being the victim of arthritis. It is too much like being taken over by decrepitude and immobility at a time in one's life when one wants and needs to be active. At the same time, and in complete opposition to this, I have done my best work, toiled for long hours, and had an immensely rewarding life, despite being a sufferer. So who am I to lapse into self-pity at having a disease which is not, after all, life-threatening, merely exceptionally inconvenient?

Many a time I have wondered whether I might have escaped RA altogether by "looking after myself" better. Certainly most books on arthritis seem to suggest that there are preventive measures one can take, such as taking regular exercise, keeping a check on one's weight, never straining or tearing joints, especially when not warmed up, and so on. They talk about keeping a good rest-activity balance, about correct posture when sitting, bending, or lifting, and about avoiding dietary extremes—all measures appropriate to the sufferer as well as to the person hoping not to become one.

Personally, I am skeptical about these preventive measures. True, they are sensible and preferable to a sluggish, overweight existence, but mine was never that anyway. I was lean, active, and sensible on every score, yet still I succumbed. In the case of my RA—and this may not be true of other conditions, such as osteoarthrosis—I do not feel that there was very much I could do to prevent it. Perhaps some of the research I discussed in the last chapter will lead future potential sufferers in a different direction.

What is clear to me is that arthritis can be fought successfully. I did so for many years while working as a heart surgeon, combined with my position as professor of cardiac surgery. In fact, I refused to give in for more than twenty years. Then I decided to give up surgery altogether. Not that my arthritis totally hampered me from performing it, but because I knew my efficiency was declining and I wanted to get out while I was ahead. Not for me the occasional small operation just to keep my hand in. Christiaan Barnard, having crossed the line as a winner once in his life, did not want to end up an also-ran. When you set yourself high standards, the important thing is to stick by them, however much grief that may cause.

After surgery, what next? Well, arthritis may be counterproductive in the operating theater, but it does not stop me from pursuing my extensive research program into tissue-rejection mechanisms, from lecturing around the world, teaching at the university, making a major television series, and of course, writing this book. This has been for me the most enjoyable part of being an arthritic, sharing the experience with you and trying to transmit that commodity I value above all others: hope. Nothing would give me more pleasure than to feel I have, at least in part, succeeded.

Bibliography

Barnard, Christiaan. *One Life*. New York: Bantam, 1971.

Dong, C. H., and Banks, J. *New Hope for the Arthritic*. London: Granada (paperback), 1983.

Dong, C. H., and Banks, J. *New Hope for the Arthritic*. London: Granada, 1980.

Dudley Hart, F. *Overcoming Arthritis*. London: Martin Dunitz, 1981.

Evans, P. *Getting On*. London: Granada, 1982.

Fairley, P. *The Conquest of Pain*. London: Michael Joseph, Ltd, 1978.

Fries, F. *Arthritis and How to Cope with It*. London: Granada, 1980.

Hooker, S. *Caring for Elderly People*. London: Routledge & Kegan Paul, 1976.

Inglis, B., and West, R. *The Alternative Health Guide*. London: Michael Joseph, Ltd, 1983.

Stanway, A. *Alternative Medicine*. London: Macdonald & Jane's, 1979.

Index

Acetaminophen (Tylenol), 50, 58, 81
Acetanilid, 51
Acetylsalicylic acid (aspirin), 50–51, 58, 81–82, 144
ACTH, 55, 59
Acupuncture, 102–7
Africans, 22, 38
Aids, 90–92
Alexander principle, 110
Allergy therapy, 124–26
Allopurinol (Lopurin, Zyloprim), 59
Alpha cure, 97
Alternative therapies, 97–113
  acupuncture, 102–7
  cellular therapy, 112–13
  homeopathy, 107–9
  hydrotherapy, 109–10
  manipulation and movement therapies, 110
  mussel extract, 111–12
  natural cures, 97–99
  psychological therapies, 110–11
American Indians, 38
Analgesics, 49–51, 58, 81–82, 143
  See also specific analgesics
Ankles, exercises for, 131–32
Ankylosing spondylitis (AS; poker back), 20, 37–40, 143–44
Antigout compounds, 59
Anti-inflammatory drugs, 82–83, 144, 145
  corticosteroids, 53–55
  nonsteroidal (NSAIDs), 51–53, 58–59
Antimalarial drugs, 55–56

Antinuclear antibody (ANA) test, 28
Antirheumatoid drugs, 56–57, 59
Anxiety, pain and, 84–85
Arthritis
  attachment, 37–41
  crystal (gout), 41–43
  definition of, 19
  miscellaneous forms of, 43–45
  osteoarthrosis, see Osteoarthrosis
  rheumatoid, see Rheumatoid arthritis
  See also specific topics
Arthritis Foundation (U.S.A.), 123–24
Arthrodesis, 74
Arthropathy, 19
Arthroplasty, 68–74
Arthrosis, 19
Aspirin (acetylsalicylic acid), 50–51, 58, 81–82, 144
Attachment arthritis, 37–41
Attitude, self-management and, 63–64
Autogenic training, 111
Autoimmune disease
  rheumatoid arthritis as, 24
  systemic lupus erythematosus, 44
Azathioprine (Imuran), 60
Azolid (phenylbutazone), 58

Back brace, belt, or corset, 81
Back pain, 106
Back surgery, 74, 75
Banks, Jane, 41
Bantu, 22
Barton, Karen, 68
Bathing, 88–89

Bathroom and dressing aids, 91
Beds, 92–93
Beecher, Henry, 78
Benemid (probenecid), 59
Biofeedback technique, 111
Blacks, 38, 40
   rheumatoid arthritis in, 22
Blaiberg, Philip, 15–16
Breathing exercises, 140
B-27 antigen test, 40
Bursae, 18
Bursitis, 44
Buskisson, Ted, 145
Butazolidin (Bute, phenylbutazone),
   51–52, 58

Calnan, J. S., 73
Capsule synovial fluid, 18
Cardiac disease, 117, 119
Cartilage, 17
   in osteoarthrosis, 30
Cellular therapy, 112–13
Cervical spondylosis, 105–6
Chairs, 88
Charnley, Sir John, 70
Charnley prosthesis, 70
Children with arthritis, 94–95
   See also Juvenile rheumatoid arthritis
Chlorambucil (Leukeran), 60
Chlordiazepoxide (Librium), 60
Chloroquine, 55–56
Chymopapain, 75
Circadian rhythm
   pain and, 79–80
   rheumatoid arthritis and, 26
Climate, rheumatoid arthritis and, 21–
   22
Clinoril (sulindac), 59
Codeine, 57, 58
Colchicine, 59
Communication, patient-doctor, 68, 70
Cooking and eating aids, 90
Corticosteroids, 53–55, 59, 145
Cortisone, 53–55
Cotswold Hills, 41
Cracciolo, Andrea, 73
Crystal arthritis (gout), 20, 41–43, 124,
   125

Crystal inflammation, 20
Cuprimine (penicillamine), 59
Cyclophosphamide (Cytoxan), 60

Dapsone, 145
Darvon (propoxyphene), 58
Debridement, 74
Degenerative disease, 20
Diazepam (Valium), 60
Dieppe, Paul, 30
Diet, 123–28
   gout and, 42
Diuretics, as precipitating factor in
   gout, 42
Dixon, A. S., 38
Dong, Collin H., 41, 124–26
DR1 factor, 23
DR4 factor, 23
Dressing, 93–94
Drinking, excessive, gout and, 42–43
Driving, 94
Drugs for treating arthritis, 47–60
   analgesics, 49–51, 58, 81–82, 143
   antigout compounds, 59
   anti-inflammatory drugs, 51–55, 82–
      83, 144, 145
   antimalarial drugs, 55–56
   antirheumatoid drugs, 56–57, 59
   corticosteroids, 53–55, 59
   immunosuppressants, 60
   nonsteroidal anti-inflammatory drugs
      (NSAIDs), 51–53, 58–59
   research on, 143–45
   tranquilizers, 60
Dudley Hart, Frank, 27, 32, 35, 79,
   83, 101–4

Eating aids, 90–91
Elbows, exercises for, 138–39
Erythrocyte sedimentation rate (ESR),
   28
Eskimos, 22
Exercise(s), 64–66, 123
   breathing, 140
   for the elbows, wrist, and hands,
      138–39
   for the feet, ankles, and knees, 131–
      33

Exercise(s) (*cont.*)
  flexibility, 128
  general, 128–29
  for the hips, 133–36
  for the shoulders and neck, 136–37
  for the spine, 129–31

Feet
  exercises for, 131–32
  replacement surgery for, 73–74
Feldenkreis technique, 110
Fenoprofen (Nalfon), 52, 59
Fibrositis, 44
Fibrous joints, 17
Finger joint replacement, 73
Flexibility exercises, 128
Freeman, Michael, 67–68, 70–72
Friedman, Meyer, 119
Fries, James F., 65, 75
Fryers, Gordon, 81
Fusion, 74

Gadgets, 90–92
Galen, 79
Gate-control theory of pain, 79
Genetics, *see* Hereditary factors
German measles (rubella), 25
Gold salts (Myochrysine), 56, 59
Gonococcus infection, 35–37
Gout (crystal arthritis), 20, 41–43, 124, 125
Grahame, Rodney, 25
Gregory, Paul, 112
Grooming, 88–89

Hallux valgus, 32
Hands, exercises for, 138–39
Heart attacks, 117, 119
Heat treatment for pain, 81
Heberden's nodes, 31
Heel, in Reiter's disease, 41
Hench, Philip S., 53
Henry VIII, King of England, 41
Hereditary factors, 13–14
  in ankylosing spondylitis, 38, 40
  in Reiter's disease, 40
  research on, 142–43
  in rheumatoid arthritis, 22–23

Hill, Alan, 49
Hip joint replacement, 68–74
Hips, exercises for the, 133–36
HLA B-27 antigen blood test, 40
HLA DRW4 antigen, 142–43
Holmes, Thomas H., 119
Homeopathy, 107–9
Hormones, osteoarthrosis and, 31
"Housemaid's knee," 44
Huskisson, 79
Hydrotherapy, 109–10
Hydroxychlorquine, 56
Hypnosis, 110–11

Ibuprofen (Motrin), 52, 58
Immobilizing a painful joint, 81
Immune system, 144–45
  rheumatoid arthritis and, 24
Immunoelectrophoresis test, 28
Immunosuppressant drugs, 57, 60
Imuran (azathioprine), 60
Indomethacin (Indocin), 52, 58
Infections
  hip replacement surgery and, 70
  Reiter's disease triggered by, 40–41
Infectious diseases of joints, 20, 35–37
Inflammatory disease, 19–20
Inglis, Brian, 110
Introversion, pain and, 83–84
Iritis, 40

Job stress, 121
Jogging, 34
Joint diseases, types of, 19–20
Joint replacements, 68–74
Joints, 17–19
Juvenile rheumatoid arthritis (JRA), 29–30, 143

Kendall, Edward C., 53
Kitchen activities, 89–90
Knee replacement operations, 68, 72–74
Knees
  exercises for, 132–33
  osteoarthrosis of, 32–33

Laboratory tests, for rheumatoid arthritis, 27–28

Latex fixation test, 28
Laying on of hands, 111
Leukeran (chlorambucil), 60
Levamisole, 145
Librium (chlordiazepoxide), 60
Ligament and tendon problems, 37–41
Ligaments, 20
Lopurin (allopurinol), 59
Lowther, Dennis, 143
Lumbago, 106
Lupus, 44–45

Madders, Jane, 120
Making love, 93
Management of arthritis, 61–66
Manipulation and movement therapies,
    110
Mann, Felix, 104–5
Mason, Maureen, 53–54
Massage, 110
Mayo Clinic, 12–13, 27
Meditation, 111
Melzack, Ronald, 79
Mental attitude, self-management and,
    63–64
6-mercaptopurine (Purinethol), 60
Metal cures, 97
Metatarsal bars, 81
Methotrexate, 60
Mobility aids, 91
Motrin (ibuprofen), 58
Muscles, inflammation of, 43
Mussel extract, 111–12
Myochrysine (gold salts), 59

Nalfon (fenoprofen), 59
Naproxen (Naprosyn), 52, 59
Natural cures, 97–99
Neck, exercises for, 137
Neck pain, 105–6
Neurological surgery, 74–75
Newell, John, 143–45, 145
Nicholls, Anne, 30–31
Niehans, Dr., 112
Nonsteroidal anti-inflammatory drugs
    (NSAIDs), 51–53, 58–59

Obesity, 126
Osteoarthritis, 19
    surgery for, 67–68
    See also Osteoarthrosis
Osteoarthrosis (OA), 19, 20, 30–35
    cartilage in, 30
    incidence and distribution of, 30–31
    primary and secondary, 34–35
    signs and symptoms of, 31–34
    x-rays in, 34
Osteophytes, 34
Osteotomy, 74
Ovens, 89
Oxalid (oxyphenbutazone), 58
Oxyphenbutazone (Oxalid, Tandearil),
    52, 58

Pain, 77–85
    anxiety and, 84–85
    as essential, 77
    gate-control theory of, 79
    heat treatment for, 81
    introversion and, 83–84
    neck, 105–6
    physical activity and, 80–81
    subjective aspects of, 78
    supports as means of controlling, 81
    threshold for, 78
    time of day (or night) and, 79–80
Painkillers (analgesics), 49–51, 81–82,
    143
Patient-doctor communication, 68, 70
Penicillamine (Cuprimine), 56–57, 59
Phenacetin, 51, 58
Phenylbutazone (Azolid; Butazolidin;
    Bute), 51–52, 58
Physical activity, 64–66
    pain and, 80–81
    See also Exercises
Podagra, 42
Poker back, see Ankylosing spondylitis
Polymyalgia rheumatica, 43
Polymyositis, 43
Prednisolone, 55, 59
Prednisone, 55, 59
Pregnancy-associated globulin (PAG),
    142

Preventive measures, 147
Probenecid (Benemid), 59
Propoxyphene (Darvon), 58
Prostheses, 68–74
Psychic healing, 111
Psychological therapies, 110–11
Purinethol (6-mercaptopurine), 60

Rahe, Richard H., 119
Recreation aids, 92
"Red light" procedure, 120
Reichstein, Tadeus, 53
Reiter's disease, 40–41
Replacement of joints, 68–74
Research, 141–46
Resection, 74
Rheumatoid arthritis, 20–30
    Dr. Barnard's personal experiences
        with, 11–16
    causes of, 24–25
    climate and, 21–22
    diagnosis of, 27
    drugs for treating, see Drugs for
        treating rheumatoid arthritis
    hereditary factors in, 22–23
    immune system and, 24
    juvenile (JRA), 29–30, 143
    laboratory tests for, 27–28
    number of people suffering from, 21
    onset of, 24
    predicting outcome of, 28–29
    rheumatoid symptoms in, 21, 22
    stress and, 22
    symptoms and signs of, 25–27
    times of day (or night) and, 25–26
    town-country disparity in, 22
    virus as cause of, 24–25
Rheumatoid factor test, 28
Rogers, Juliet, 30
Rolfing, 110
Rosenberg, Jeffrey, 143–44
Rosenman, Roy, 119
Rubella (German measles), 25
Rubens, Peter Paul, 22
Rural dwellers, rheumatoid arthritis in,
    22

Sacroiliac joints, in ankylosing spondy-
    litis, 38, 40
Salicylates, 50–51
Salsburg, Richard, 144
Sciatica, 75, 106
Sedimentation rate test, 40, 43
Self-management, 61–66
Sex, 93
Shoulders, exercises for, 136–37
Sitting, 88
Sleeping, 92
Slipped spinal disk, 106
    chympopapain treatment for, 75
Social readjustment scale, 118, 119
Spine, exercises for the, 129–31
Splint, 81
Staphylococcus (staph) infections, 35,
    36
Steere, Allen, 143
Steroids, 144, 145
Still's disease, 29
Still, G. F., 29
Stoves, 89
Stress, 115–22
    personal experiences of Dr. Barnard
        with, 115–17, 119, 121
    rheumatoid arthritis and, 22
Structural Integration, 110
Sulindac (Clinoril), 52, 59
Surgical treatments, 67–76
    cosmetic benefits of, 75
    foot joint replacement, 73–74
    hip joint replacement, 68–74
    knee joint replacement, 68, 72–74
    neurological, 74–75
    for osteoarthritis, 67–68
    for osteoarthrosis-type conditions, 74
    patient-doctor communication and,
        68, 70
    personal experience of Dr. Barnard
        with, 75–76
Synovectomy, 74
Synovial membrane, 18
Synovitis, 19–28
Systemic lupus erythematosus, 44–45

Tandearil (oxyphenbutazone), 58

Tendon problems, 20
Tendons, 18
Tests for rheumatoid arthritis, 27
Tissue-type factors, in rheumatoid arthritis, 23
Tolmetin (Tolectin), 52, 59
Total complement test, 28
Tranquilizers, 60
Triamcinolone hexacetonide, 59
Trick movements, 89
Tuberculosis, 35, 37
Tylenol (acetaminophen), 58
Type A personality, 119–20

Urban dwellers, rheumatoid arthritis in, 22
Urethritis, 37
Uric acid, 42–43

Valium (diazepam), 60
Venereal disease, 35–37

Walking sticks, 91
Wall, Patrick, 79
Watt, Iain, 30
Weight, 126, 127
Weight-control diet, 126, 128
West, Ruth, 110
Wingate, Peter, 53, 55
Woodrow, John, 23
Workplace, stress in, 121
Wright, Verna, 68
Wrist, exercises for, 138–39

X-rays, 28
    in ankylosing spondylitis, 40
    in osteoarthrosis, 34

Yoga, 110

Zyloprim (allopurinol), 59